First, Do No Harm

First, Do No Harm

Building a Sustainable Health Care Future with AI and Digital Technologies

Rubin Pillay MD, PhD

Copyright © 2024 by Rubin Pillay MD, PhD.

Library of Congress Control Number:		2024923310
ISBN:	Hardcover	979-8-3694-3202-0
	Softcover	979-8-3694-3201-3
	eBook	979-8-3694-3200-6

All rights reserved. No part of this book may be reproduced or transmitted in any form or by any means, electronic or mechanical, including photocopying, recording, or by any information storage and retrieval system, without permission in writing from the copyright owner.

Any people depicted in stock imagery provided by Getty Images are models, and such images are being used for illustrative purposes only. Certain stock imagery © Getty Images.

Print information available on the last page.

Rev. date: 10/29/2024

To order additional copies of this book, contact:
Xlibris
844-714-8691
www.Xlibris.com
Orders@Xlibris.com
862938

Contents

Preface vii

Chapter 1   Health Care's Climate Footprint: An Inconvenient Truth ... 1
Chapter 2   Digitalization and Environmental Sustainability 13
Chapter 3   Digital Health Trends and Their Material Footprint 34
Chapter 4   Environmental Impacts in the Use Phase of Digital Health Technologies 53
Chapter 5   The End-of-Life Challenge: Managing Digital Health Waste 76
Chapter 6   Digital Health Platforms and Environmental Sustainability 101
Chapter 7   Toward Environmentally Sustainable Digital Health that Works for Inclusive Health Care 128
Chapter 8   Policy Options for Environmentally Sustainable Digital Development 150

Conclusion 155
About the Author 159

Preface

The rapid digitalization of health care continues at an unprecedented pace, transforming how we deliver care, manage health systems, and interact with patients. While this digital revolution offers immense potential to improve health outcomes and increase access to care, it also presents significant challenges that must be carefully addressed to ensure we uphold our fundamental principle as health care providers: First, do no harm.

This book, *First Do No Harm: Building a Sustainable Health Care Future with AI and Digital Technologies*, explores the critical intersection of health care digitalization and environmental sustainability. As we embrace artificial intelligence, telemedicine, electronic health records, and other digital innovations, we must also confront the environmental impact of these technologies—from the depletion of raw materials and increased energy consumption to the generation of electronic waste.

The health care sector already has a substantial environmental footprint, estimated to be responsible for 4.4 percent of global net emissions. As we integrate more digital technologies, we risk exacerbating our impact on climate change and environmental degradation, unless we take a thoughtful, sustainable approach.

Yet digitalization also offers unprecedented opportunities to make health care more efficient, effective, and environmentally friendly. AI and digital tools can optimize resource use, reduce unnecessary treatments and travel, and enable innovative solutions for both improving patient care and mitigating our climate impact.

This book calls for a balanced, holistic approach to health care digitalization—one that harnesses the immense potential of technology to advance health equity and improve outcomes, while simultaneously minimizing negative environmental impacts. We must strive for a circular digital health care economy, characterized by responsible consumption, renewable energy use, and comprehensive management of electronic medical waste.

As we navigate this complex landscape, collaboration across the health care ecosystem is paramount. From policymakers and hospital administrators to clinicians, technologists, and patients, we all have a role to play in shaping an environmentally sustainable and inclusive digital health future.

The choices we make today in implementing digital health technologies will have far-reaching consequences for both human and planetary health. This book aims to provide valuable insights and recommendations for all stakeholders committed to building a health care system that leverages the power of digitalization while safeguarding the well-being of our planet and future generations.

Let us seize this opportunity to create a digital health care economy that not only improves patient outcomes but also thrives in harmony with our environment. The health of our patients and the health of our planet are inextricably linked—it's time our approach to health care innovation reflects this fundamental truth.

Chapter 1

Health Care's Climate Footprint: An Inconvenient Truth

In a paradoxical twist, the very sector dedicated to safeguarding human health is contributing significantly to the greatest health threat of the twenty-first century—climate change. The global health care industry, with its mission to protect and promote well-being, finds itself in the uncomfortable position of being a major contributor to the climate crisis it aims to mitigate.

The scale of health care's environmental impact is staggering. According to recent studies, the sector's global climate footprint is equivalent to a staggering 4.4 percent of global net emissions, amounting to 2 gigatons of carbon dioxide equivalent annually. To put this into perspective, if the health sector were a country, it would rank as the fifth-largest emitter on the planet. This carbon footprint is comparable to the annual greenhouse gas emissions from 514 coal-fired power plants.

As we delve deeper into health care's climate impact, we must confront this inconvenient truth: The industry tasked with healing is inadvertently harming the very environment that sustains us all. This realization underscores the urgent need for the health care sector to play a pivotal role in addressing the climate crisis, not just as a responder to its health impacts but also as a leader in reducing its own substantial environmental footprint.

1.1 Top Health Care Emitters: A Global Perspective

The global distribution of health care–related emissions reveals stark disparities among nations, reflecting differences in health care systems, economic development, and population size. This analysis provides crucial insights into where the most significant opportunities for emission reductions lie.

United States: The Leading Emitter

The United States stands out as the world's largest health care emitter, both in absolute terms and per capita. Its health care sector produces a staggering fifty-seven times more emissions per person than India. This disproportionate contribution underscores the urgent need for the U.S. health care system to prioritize sustainability and emission reduction strategies.

China and the European Union: Significant Contributors

China and the collective countries of the European Union, along with the United States, account for more than half (56 percent) of the world's total health care climate footprint. This concentration of emissions in just three regions highlights the potential impact of targeted interventions in these areas.

Top Ten Emitters: A Global Responsibility

The top ten health care emitters collectively contribute 75 percent of the global health care climate footprint. This concentration suggests that focused efforts on these countries could yield significant reductions in overall health care–related emissions.

Disparities in Per Capita Emissions

While absolute numbers are important, per capita emissions reveal interesting patterns:

- India, despite having the seventh-largest absolute health care sector climate footprint, has the lowest health-related emissions per capita among the 43 nations studied in detail.
- China's health care sector produces six times more greenhouse gases per person than India's. However, it still emits only one-seventh of the greenhouse gases per capita compared to the United States, one-third that of Korea, and just under half of the European Union's per capita emissions.

These disparities highlight the complex relationship between health care provision, population size, and emissions. They also point to the potential for high-emitting countries to learn from more efficient systems in lower-emitting nations.

1.2 Implications for Global Health and Climate Policy

The concentration of emissions in a handful of countries presents both a challenge and an opportunity. While it underscores the outsized impact of certain health care systems on global emissions, it also suggests that targeted interventions in these high-emitting countries could have a significant impact on reducing the overall health care climate footprint.

Moreover, the vast differences in per capita emissions between countries like the United States and India indicate that it's possible to provide health care with a much lower carbon footprint. This realization should spur global innovation and knowledge sharing among health care systems, aiming to combine high-quality care with environmental sustainability.

As we move forward in addressing the climate crisis, it's clear that the health care sectors of the world's largest emitters must take a leading role in reducing their environmental impact. Simultaneously, emerging health care systems in developing nations have the opportunity to leapfrog to more sustainable models, avoiding the high-emission pathways of their predecessors.

1.3 Sources of Health Care's Climate Footprint

The health care sector's contribution to climate change is complex and multifaceted, with emissions stemming from various sources across its operations and supply chain. Understanding these sources is crucial for developing effective strategies to reduce the sector's environmental impact.

Health care facilities contribute to greenhouse gas emissions through both direct and indirect means. *Scope 1 emissions*—direct emissions from health care facilities and vehicles owned by health care organizations—account for 17 percent of total emissions. These include on-site fuel combustion for heating and power generation as well as anesthetic gases.

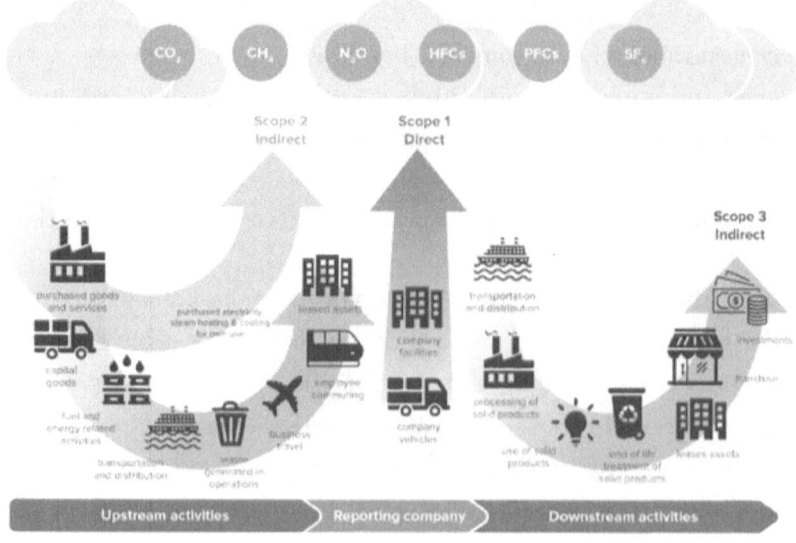

Scope 2 emissions arise from purchased energy sources like electricity and heating, comprising another 12 percent of total emissions. However, a staggering 71 percent of health care's climate footprint comes from *Scope 3 emissions*, primarily derived from its supply chain through activities such as the production, transport, and disposal of pharmaceuticals and medical devices.

Interestingly, approximately 75 percent of all health care emissions are generated domestically within the country where services are consumed. This indicates that while health care's impact is global, a significant portion can be addressed through local initiatives.

At the heart of these emissions lies fossil fuel consumption. Energy use—primarily from fossil fuel combustion—makes up well over half of health care's total climate footprint across all three scopes. This underscores the critical importance of transitioning to renewable energy sources and improving energy efficiency in health care settings.

Understanding these sources of emissions is crucial for developing targeted strategies to reduce health care's climate impact.

The following are among the key areas for action:

1. Improving energy efficiency and transitioning to renewable energy sources in health care facilities
2. Optimizing transportation and logistics in health care operations
3. Implementing sustainable procurement practices to address supply-chain emissions
4. Developing and adopting low-carbon medical technologies and pharmaceuticals

By addressing the key sources of emissions, the health care sector can significantly reduce its climate footprint while continuing to provide high-quality care. This not only aligns with the sector's mission to protect health, but it also positions health care as a leader in the global fight against climate change.

1.4 Health Care's Footprint: The Spending-Emissions Nexus

The relationship between a country's health care spending and its climate footprint is complex and multifaceted. Research has revealed a strong, though not absolute, correlation between these two factors. Generally, countries that allocate a higher percentage of their GDP to health care tend to have higher per capita health care emissions.

This correlation raises important questions about the sustainability of health care systems as they expand and improve. As nations strive to enhance their health care services and work toward goals like universal health coverage, they must also grapple with the environmental implications of these advancements.

However, it's crucial to note that health care spending is not the sole determinant of a sector's climate footprint. Other factors play critical roles in shaping the environmental impact of health care systems. These are two particularly significant factors:

1. The energy intensity of a country's economy

    This refers to how much energy is used to produce a unit of economic output. Countries with more energy-intensive economies tend to have higher emissions across all sectors, including health care.

2. The emissions intensity of a country's energy system

    This relates to the amount of greenhouse gases emitted per unit of energy produced. Countries relying heavily on fossil fuels for energy production will have higher emissions in their health care sector and beyond.

These factors highlight the interconnected nature of health care emissions with broader economic and energy policies. They also point to potential avenues for reducing health care's climate footprint without compromising on the quality or accessibility of care.

The path forward lies in decoupling health care spending from emissions growth. If the health sector's growth and investment can be coupled with a trajectory toward zero emissions, it's possible to significantly decrease health care's climate footprint even as health spending increases. This approach could create a win-win scenario, allowing countries to pursue health sector development goals such as universal health coverage while simultaneously working toward global climate targets.

Achieving this decoupling will require innovative approaches across the health care system. These might include the following:

- investing in energy-efficient medical technologies and facilities
- transitioning to renewable energy sources for health care operations
- implementing sustainable procurement practices in medical supply chains
- promoting telemedicine and other low-carbon models of care delivery

By adopting such strategies, the health care sector can lead by example in the fight against climate change. It can demonstrate that it's possible to improve human health and well-being while also safeguarding the health of our planet.

As we move forward, policymakers, health care leaders, and environmental experts must work together to develop strategies that allow for the expansion and improvement of health care services without proportionally increasing the sector's environmental impact. This balanced approach is crucial for creating a health care system that is not only effective and accessible but also sustainable in the long term.

1.5 The Health Sector's Responsibility: Addressing Its Climate Footprint

As the global community grapples with the escalating climate crisis, the health care sector finds itself in a unique position. Not only must it respond to the health impacts of climate change, it must also confront its own significant contribution to the problem. This dual responsibility presents both a challenge and an opportunity for the sector to lead by example in the fight against climate change.

- Responding to the Climate Emergency

The health sector's primary role in addressing the climate crisis has traditionally been reactive—treating those who fall ill, suffer injuries, or face mortality due to climate-related events and their underlying causes. However, this approach is no longer sufficient. The sector must now embrace a proactive stance, focusing on primary prevention by actively working to mitigate the root cause of these health issues: climate change itself.

This shift toward prevention requires a radical reduction in the sector's own emissions. By doing so, health care can directly contribute to slowing climate change and indirectly reduce the future burden of climate-related illnesses and injuries.

- Aligning with Global Climate Goals

To truly make a difference, the health care sector's climate action must align with the ambitious targets set by the Paris Agreement. This means working toward achieving net zero emissions by 2050 or earlier. Such a goal requires a comprehensive approach that extends beyond individual health care facilities to encompass entire health systems, ministries of health, and, crucially, the entire supply chain of health care goods and services.

Achieving this level of decarbonization will require unprecedented collaboration between health care providers, policymakers, and manufacturers. It will involve reimagining everything from the energy sources powering hospitals to the materials used in medical devices and the transportation methods for delivering health care services.

- Balancing Climate Action with Health Care Goals

The challenge for the health care sector lies in pursuing aggressive climate action while simultaneously working toward other critical objectives. These include achieving universal health coverage and meeting the United Nations' Sustainable Development Goals. This balancing act requires innovative thinking and strategic planning to ensure that efforts to reduce emissions do not come at the cost of health care quality or accessibility.

In fact, many climate-friendly initiatives can also improve health care delivery and access. For instance, investments in telemedicine can both reduce travel-related emissions and increase access to care in remote areas. Similarly, energy-efficient hospitals can lower operating costs, potentially freeing up resources for expanded services.

- Leading by Example

Encouragingly, several health systems across multiple countries are already pioneering the way toward decarbonization. These trailblazers serve as vital models for the rest of the sector, demonstrating that significant emissions reductions are not only possible but can also be achieved while maintaining, or even improving, the quality of care.

For example:

- The National Health Service (NHS) in England has committed to reaching net zero emissions by 2040 for the emissions it directly controls, and by 2045 for those it can influence.

- Kaiser Permanente, a large U.S. health care provider, became carbon neutral in 2020, primarily through investments in renewable energy and energy efficiency.
- Hospitals in India and Costa Rica have implemented solar power systems, significantly reducing their reliance on fossil fuels.

These examples show that with commitment, innovation, and strategic planning, health care organizations can make substantial progress in reducing their climate footprint.

1.6 Climate Change Is a Health Issue

Climate change is increasingly recognized as a significant health issue, affecting human health today and posing even greater risks in the future. *The Lancet* has labeled it the "biggest global health threat of the 21st century," highlighting the urgency of addressing its impacts. Direct consequences of climate change, such as the spread of vector-borne diseases, rising temperatures, droughts, severe storms, and flooding, are already evident and will intensify over time. These effects disproportionately impact vulnerable and marginalized populations, exacerbating existing health disparities. All countries will experience significant health impacts from climate change, but low- and middle-income nations will bear the brunt of these effects due to their heightened vulnerability and limited capacity to adapt, often characterized by weak health systems and inadequate infrastructure. It is estimated that climate change could push more than 100 million people back into extreme poverty by 2030, with many of these reversals linked to adverse health outcomes.

The Lancet Countdown on health and climate warns that the lack of progress in reducing emissions and enhancing adaptive capacity threatens not only human lives but also the viability of national health systems. This situation has the potential to disrupt essential public health infrastructure and overwhelm health care services. Hospitals, health centers, and public health workers are on the front lines, responding to the health effects of climate change. As extreme climate events become more frequent and severe, health care systems will incur substantial costs and must develop resilience against these impacts. Unfortunately, some of the world's poorest health systems are also among the most vulnerable, lacking both resources and tools to effectively protect their populations.

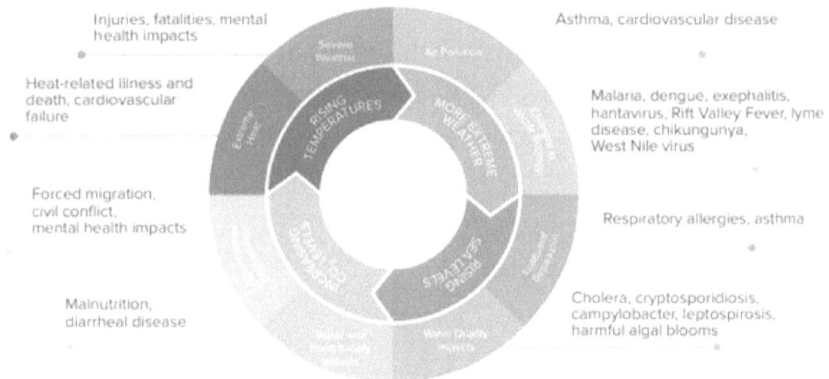

Moreover, fossil fuel combustion—the primary driver of climate change—contributes significantly to current health problems. Air pollution from fossil fuels is responsible for over 7 million premature deaths each year, roughly twice as many as those caused by HIV/AIDS, malaria, and tuberculosis combined. Additionally, air pollution is a major contributor to chronic diseases that require treatment and hospitalization, leading to increased health care spending and emissions. This burden falls disproportionately on low- and middle-income countries, where over 80 percent of premature deaths attributed to non-communicable diseases occur.

Despite these challenges, there is a significant opportunity for prevention. The worst effects and causes of climate change can be mitigated through proactive measures that not only address environmental issues but also improve health outcomes and promote equity in health care access. By recognizing climate change as a critical health issue, health care professionals can advocate for sustainable practices that protect both public health and the environment. This dual approach can lead to a healthier population while simultaneously combating one of the most pressing challenges of our time.

The health care sector's responsibility in addressing climate change is clear and urgent. By taking decisive action to reduce its own emissions, the sector can play a crucial role in mitigating the climate crisis while continuing to fulfill its primary mission of protecting and improving human health. As more health care organizations join this effort, the sector has the potential to become a powerful force for positive change, demonstrating that it's possible to provide high-quality care while also safeguarding the health of our planet.

Chapter 2

Digitalization and Environmental Sustainability

2.1 The Health Care Digitalization and Environmental Sustainability Nexus

As the digital revolution in health care continues to create both unprecedented opportunities and complex challenges for patient care and health system sustainability, this chapter turns our attention to a critical yet often overlooked aspect: the environmental implications of health care AI and digitalization. The promise of artificial intelligence (AI) and digital technologies to transform patient care, improve health outcomes, and increase access to health services is undeniable. However, as we embrace these innovations, we must also confront a new dimension of our fundamental principle: "First, do no harm."

Against a backdrop of escalating climate change and its profound impacts on global health, digital solutions are increasingly being leveraged to address environmental health risks and improve care delivery. However, it is equally crucial to consider how we can reduce the environmental footprint of health care digitalization itself.

This chapter outlines the importance of exploring the intricate relationship between health care digitalization and environmental sustainability. We stress the need to consider the entire life cycle of digital health products and systems—from the raw materials used in medical devices to the energy consumption of data centers storing electronic health records and the disposal of obsolete health care technology.

We also highlight a particular challenge faced by many developing countries and underserved health care systems. These regions often lack the resources to fully harness digital health technologies for improving care and mitigating environmental health risks. Simultaneously, they may bear a disproportionate burden of the environmental costs associated with health care digitalization, such as electronic waste disposal or resource extraction.

By examining these complex dynamics, this chapter sets the stage for a comprehensive exploration of how we can build a more sustainable digital health future—one that improves patient outcomes, enhances health system efficiency, and minimizes negative environmental impacts.

2.2 Redefining "First, Do No Harm" for the Digital Age

The Hippocratic oath, taken by physicians for centuries, has long been the cornerstone of medical ethics. However, in the age of digital health, we must expand our understanding of harm to include environmental impacts. The health care sector, while dedicated to healing, paradoxically contributes significantly to environmental degradation and climate change, accounting for approximately 4.4 percent of global net emissions.

The rapid digitalization of health care, while offering immense benefits, has largely overlooked its environmental footprint. From the energy-intensive production of medical devices to the power consumption of data centers hosting electronic health records, the environmental costs are substantial yet often hidden.

Balancing patient care with planetary health presents a complex challenge. As we strive to provide the best possible care through advanced technologies, we must also consider the long-term environmental impacts of our choices. This requires a paradigm shift in how we approach health care delivery, emphasizing sustainability alongside efficacy and efficiency.

2.3 The Intersection of Digital Health and Environmental Sustainability

Sustainable health care is a vital priority for global health organizations and the medical community, articulated in numerous international health conferences and in the United Nations' Sustainable Development Goals. Sustainable health care implies delivering high-quality care that meets current health needs without compromising the ability of future generations to meet their own health needs. This concept aligns with the protection of planetary boundaries and intergenerational equity in health care delivery.

In this context, three issues have become critical in health care: the consumption of medical resources, the impact of climate change on health, and medical waste and pollution. The cost of failure in these areas threatens not only the sustainability of health care systems but also global public health.

The World Health Organization has urged all stakeholders—governments, health care providers, and civil society—to recognize that environmental protection must be an integral part of health care delivery and cannot be considered in isolation. Consequently, health care practices that are not environmentally sustainable will ultimately prove unsustainable for human health.

Recent advancements in digital health technologies have profoundly impacted health care delivery, offering potential for more inclusive and sustainable practices. These technologies, including artificial intelligence, telemedicine, and electronic health records, are rapidly changing the nature of health care. However, they also bring challenges, including widening digital health divides and significant environmental implications.

The digital transformation of health care is occurring alongside growing concerns about resource depletion, energy use, and medical waste generation. Managing this digital transformation will greatly influence both the future of health care and environmental health. This report explores the interconnectedness of rapid health care digitalization and the urgent need to foster environmental sustainability against a backdrop of growing health inequities and environmental vulnerabilities.

The topic is timely and overdue, as discussions on environmental sustainability and digital health have been evolving separately for too long. Major global health initiatives and agreements have often failed to fully recognize the relationship between digital health technologies and environmental sustainability.

For instance, while the UN Sustainable Development Goals emphasize health and well-being, they do not take a cross-cutting view of the role of digital health. Similarly, international climate agreements often highlight digital technologies as tools for sharing health information and improving health care efficiency without fully considering their direct environmental impact.

Digital health continues to evolve rapidly, offering new solutions for health care delivery but also presenting new challenges for sustainability. The relationship between digital health and environmental sustainability is starting to receive more attention in health policy debates, with a focus on maximizing the benefits of digital health while mitigating its environmental harm.

There are growing references to "twin transitions" in health care—the shift toward more digital systems and the move toward more environmentally sustainable practices. These transitions are closely intertwined within the broader evolution of global health systems. Environmentally sustainable health care needs digital tools to become more efficient and resilient, while digital health solutions need to be as environmentally sustainable as possible to avoid exacerbating health risks.

Moreover, the resources needed for digital health technologies and for addressing climate change–related health issues are often the same, creating competing demands and influencing global health dynamics.

It's crucial to ensure that no one is left behind as we transition toward a more digital and environmentally sustainable health care future. This requires an integrated approach that balances improved health outcomes, environmental protection, and economic viability within a framework of ethical governance and health equity.

The intersection of digital health and environmental sustainability needs considerably more attention. We must examine how the rapidly evolving digital health landscape impacts environmental sustainability and what this means for global health equity and development. Addressing these complex, interrelated challenges is essential for building a truly sustainable health care system for the future.

2.4 The Rapidly Evolving Nature of Digital Health

When assessing the intersection of digital health and environmental sustainability, it's crucial to acknowledge the dynamic nature of health care technologies and their applications. The continuous evolution of digital health creates new opportunities for leveraging data and technologies to improve patient care and mitigate adverse health and environmental impacts. Simultaneously, ensuring the environmental sustainability of digital health ecosystems becomes increasingly important.

- Higher-speed connectivity: Accelerated progress in high-speed internet has opened up opportunities for new digital health applications, such as telemedicine, remote patient monitoring, and AI-powered diagnostics. The digital delivery of health care

services relies on greater bandwidth to support high-quality video consultations and medical imaging transfers. However, access to these opportunities still varies greatly across different regions.
- Shift to cloud-based health records: Cloud computing is transforming health care data management. It enables health care providers to access scalable and flexible storage for electronic health records (EHRs) and medical imaging. While the "cloud" imagery suggests intangibility, cloud-based health systems are anchored in physical data centers, often controlled by a small number of large tech companies.
- Health platform expansion: Digital health platforms, acting as intermediaries, are uniquely positioned to capture and analyze extensive patient data. Their expansion is linked to their capacity to collect, analyze, and potentially monetize health data, ranging from fitness tracking to complex medical diagnostics. This trend has led to market concentration dominated by a few global digital health platforms.
- Exponential health data growth: The surge in digital health tool usage has significantly boosted interconnectedness among patients, health care providers, and medical devices. Real-time data generated from improved interconnectedness can help address various health challenges, including chronic disease management and epidemic response. The Internet of Medical Things (IoMT) is expected to expand rapidly, employing various devices to collect and transmit timely health data.
- AI in health care: The exponential increase in health data generation is amplifying the importance of big data analytics, machine learning, and AI in health care. Global investment in health care AI has surged dramatically in recent years. While offering new diagnostic and treatment possibilities, AI applications in health care are computationally costly, energy-intensive, and generate significant electronic waste.
- Virtual and augmented reality in medicine: These technologies offer new possibilities in medical training, surgical planning, and patient education. While they can enhance medical care and potentially

reduce the need for physical resources, their environmental impact depends on the inputs required and whether they replace or complement existing medical practices.
- Blockchain in health care: Distributed ledger technologies hold the potential for secure health data management, drug traceability, and streamlined insurance claims processing. However, some blockchain applications, particularly those using proof-of-work mechanisms, demand significant computational resources and energy.

As these digital health technologies continue to evolve and expand, their environmental implications will depend on adoption rates, efficiency improvements, and conscious efforts to balance health benefits with sustainability concerns.

2.5 Comprehensive Life Cycle Assessments in Digital Health

The relationship between digital health and environmental sustainability is multifaceted and can be explored from various perspectives. There's a growing need to consider how digital health technologies comply with "planetary health boundaries" related to climate, biodiversity, and resource use. Key environmental impacts of digital health are linked to energy use, greenhouse gas (GHG) emissions, water consumption, and electronic waste generation. These impacts are closely tied to the concept of the Anthropocene, reflecting how human activity, including health care practices, has a long-lasting impact on the environment.

Digital health solutions are often seen as key to achieving sustainable development goals in health care, such as improving health outcomes while reducing resource consumption. For example, they can potentially reduce the environmental impacts of health care delivery through telemedicine, AI-powered diagnostics, and enhanced operational efficiency. This raises a critical question of how to better leverage digital health to achieve sustainability in health care, for which improved data and measuring approaches are needed.

Hence, the main focus of this discussion is how to make digital health technologies and activities more sustainable. Unless adequately addressed, their negative environmental impacts are likely to increase as digital health expands across all areas of health care delivery.

Discussions of sustainable health care have increasingly focused on the desirability of a more circular economy to reduce environmental impacts. Most medical devices and digital health technologies today are produced in an essentially linear model, from raw material extraction to disposal. A more circular digital health economy would seek to reduce, reuse, and recycle medical devices and digital health infrastructure, including by extending their lifespan. This can be achieved through sharing, maintenance and repair, resale and redistribution, as well as remanufacturing and refurbishing medical equipment and devices.

To better understand these impacts, researchers use life-cycle assessments (LCAs) to evaluate the environmental impacts of digital health products or services throughout their entire life span. LCA in digital health is not limited to any single environmental indicator, such as greenhouse gas (GHG) emissions but can encompass multiple criteria including resource depletion, water use, and toxic emissions.

For digital health transformation, LCA can help to identify stages with important environmental impact from medical devices, health IT infrastructure, and data centers. It can highlight potential environmental trade-offs and assess the sustainability potential of substituting digital for traditional health care technologies.

This assessment examines three phases of the life cycle of digital health technologies:

1. The *production phase* covers the extraction of raw materials for medical devices and health IT infrastructure, their manufacturing,

and global distribution. This phase is particularly important when considering the intensity of rare earth mineral use in many medical devices.
2. The *use phase* considers environmental effects generated by operating and using digital health technologies, including energy use, GHG emissions, and water consumption by data centers hosting health records and running AI algorithms.
3. The *end-of-life phase* looks at the treatment of digital health technologies after use and the importance of moving toward a more circular economy in health care technology.

By applying comprehensive life-cycle assessments to digital health technologies, we can better understand their full environmental impact and develop strategies to minimize any negative effects while maximizing health benefits. This holistic approach is crucial for ensuring that the digital transformation of health care contributes positively to both human and planetary health.

2.6 Direct and Indirect Effects of Digital Health Technologies

To assess the overall environmental impact of digital health, it's crucial to distinguish between direct and indirect effects across the life cycle of health care technologies.

A. Direct Effects

Direct effects result from digital health devices and infrastructure throughout their lifecycle, from raw material extraction to end-of-life disposal. These effects constitute the "environmental footprint" of digital health and include the following:

- Resource use: Production of medical devices and health IT infrastructure requires significant resources, including rare earth minerals.

- Energy consumption: Operation of medical equipment, data centers storing health records, and AI systems for diagnostics consume substantial energy.
- GHG emissions: Both production and use of digital health technologies contribute to greenhouse gas emissions.
- Water usage: Significant amounts of water are used in manufacturing processes and for cooling data centers hosting health information.
- E-waste generation: Rapid obsolescence of medical devices and health IT equipment contributes to electronic waste.

It's important to consider impacts beyond just GHG emissions. For instance, the extraction of raw materials for medical devices can impact biodiversity and cause soil contamination.

B. Indirect and Rebound Effects

Indirect effects describe the broader environmental impacts of using digital health technologies across the health care sector. These can be both beneficial and harmful:

Positive indirect effects ("enabling effects"):

- Telemedicine reduces patient travel and associated emissions
- AI optimizes resource use in hospitals, reducing energy consumption and waste
- Digital health records will reduce paper waste.

However, these potential gains may be counterbalanced by "rebound effects":

- Improved health care access through digital tools may increase overall health care consumption.
- Time saved through digital health efficiencies might be used for other resource-intensive activities.
- Lowered skill thresholds for certain medical tasks (e.g., AI-assisted diagnostics) may increase their frequency.

Even if digital health achieves efficiency improvements, behavioral changes and increased overall health care consumption may mitigate anticipated environmental benefits.

C. Uncertain Combined Effects of Digital Health

Understanding the cumulative environmental effects of digital health is crucial. The net impact depends on whether digital health is considered part of the problem or part of the solution for environmental sustainability in health care:

- Direct negative impacts arise from the production, use, and disposal of digital health devices and infrastructure.
- The indirect effects of applying digital technologies in health care can be both positive (e.g., optimizing resource use) and negative (e.g., inducing more health care consumption).
- Systemic effects due to behavioral or structural changes in health care delivery can either reduce or increase environmental impact.

The indirect environmental effects of digital health could potentially be significantly greater than the direct footprint. For example, the emissions saved by avoiding patient travel through telemedicine might far outweigh the emissions from running the telemedicine system. However, if telemedicine leads to more frequent consultations overall, the net effect becomes more complex to assess.

Challenges in measuring indirect effects often lead to their exclusion when assessing the true environmental impact of digital health. This underlines the importance of developing better standardized frameworks to account for these effects in health care technology assessment.

Regardless of indirect impacts, minimizing the direct environmental footprint of digital health technologies remains essential. As the health care sector continues to digitalize, understanding and mitigating both direct and indirect environmental effects will be crucial for building a truly sustainable health system.

2.7 Opportunities for Digital Health Technologies to Mitigate Carbon Emissions in Health Care

Digital health technologies offer significant potential to reduce the environmental impact of health care delivery across various areas. While empirical evidence on actual gains remains limited in many cases, this section explores potential opportunities for environmental sustainability in health care through digital innovation.

- Electronic Health Records (EHRs) and Telemedicine

EHRs can significantly reduce paper waste and associated carbon emissions from the production and disposal of physical medical records. Telemedicine, by reducing the need for patient travel, can potentially decrease transportation-related emissions. A study by the University of California Davis Health System found that their telemedicine program could reduce carbon dioxide emissions by 1,969 metric tons annually, equivalent to taking 424 passenger vehicles off the road for a year.

- AI-Powered Diagnostics and Treatment Planning

Artificial Intelligence can optimize diagnostic processes, potentially reducing unnecessary tests and their associated environmental impacts. For instance, AI-assisted image analysis could reduce the need for repeat scans, lowering energy consumption and radiation exposure. AI can also help in treatment planning, potentially reducing resource waste from ineffective treatments.

- Smart Hospitals and the Internet of Medical Things

Smart building technologies in hospitals can optimize energy use through automated lighting, heating, and cooling systems. The Internet of Medical

Things can improve equipment tracking and utilization, reducing unnecessary purchases and associated manufacturing emissions. One study estimated that smart hospital solutions could reduce a hospital's carbon footprint by up to 50 percent.

- Precision Medicine and Personalized Health Care

Digital health technologies enabling precision medicine can potentially reduce medication waste by ensuring patients receive the most effective treatments based on their genetic profile. This could decrease the environmental impact of pharmaceutical production and disposal.

- Supply Chain Optimization

Digital technologies can enhance the sustainability of health care supply chains by optimizing logistics, reducing overstock and waste, and improving the tracking of medical supplies. Blockchain technology, for instance, could improve the traceability of pharmaceuticals, potentially reducing counterfeit drugs and associated waste.

- Remote Patient Monitoring

Continuous remote monitoring of chronic conditions can potentially reduce hospital admissions and associated resource use. A study in the UK found that telehealth services for chronic obstructive pulmonary disease patients reduced hospital admissions by 20 percent, which could translate to significant reductions in health care-related emissions.

- 3D Printing in Health Care

The 3D printing of medical devices and implants can potentially reduce manufacturing waste and transportation emissions associated with traditional production methods. It also allows for on-demand production, potentially reducing overstock and associated waste.

- Digital Health Education:

Digital platforms for medical education and training can reduce the need for travel to conferences and training sessions, potentially decreasing associated carbon emissions.

While these digital health technologies offer promising opportunities for reducing health care's carbon footprint, it's important to note that their implementation also carries environmental costs. The production, use, and disposal of digital health devices and infrastructure have their own environmental impacts. Therefore, a holistic approach considering both the benefits and the environmental costs of digital health technologies is crucial for achieving true sustainability in health care.

As the health care sector continues to digitalize, further research and real-world implementation studies will be vital to quantify the actual environmental benefits of these technologies and to develop strategies for maximizing their positive impact while minimizing potential negative effects.

2.8 Assessing the overall direct environmental footprint of AI and Digital Health

Accurately assessing the direct environmental impacts of digital health technologies is challenging. The rapid evolution of health care technologies and changing practices complicate measurement, with numerous factors affecting environmental impacts, such as resource depletion, GHG emissions, water consumption, and e-waste generation. Taking a broad, multi-criteria perspective on the environmental footprint, available research suggests that the production phase of medical devices and health IT infrastructure has the greatest impact. This is due to mineral and metal depletion, GHG emissions generated, and water-related impacts. During the use phase, the energy consumption of medical equipment and data centers and associated GHG emissions are the main concerns.

2.8.1 Measurement Challenges in Health Care Technology

Comprehensive assessments of the environmental footprint of digital health are scarce due to several factors:

- Data scarcity: There's a lack of timely, comparable, and accessible data regarding the energy and environmental impacts of digital health technologies. No harmonized reporting standards exist, and there's often limited disclosure of impacts such as effects on local watersheds.
- Scope variation: The scope of what constitutes "digital health" varies between studies. Some may include only electronic health records and telemedicine systems, while others might encompass AI-powered diagnostic tools, wearable devices, and IoT medical sensors.
- Life-cycle stage definitions: Studies vary in how they define the life-cycle stages of digital health technologies. While some standards exist (e.g., ISO 14040 for Life Cycle Assessment), they are not consistently followed in health care technology research.
- Methodological differences: Even studies looking at similar life-cycle stages reach different conclusions due to varying assumptions and models used to estimate environmental impact. For example, variations include the anticipated growth of digital health adoption, its correlation with energy consumption, and the extent to which digital health will contribute to emissions reductions in other areas of health care.
- Global vs. local impact: Most studies position themselves as global analyses. However, the environmental impacts of digital health can have varying effects at local, regional, and global levels. For instance, the production of medical devices might have localized impacts on water quality in manufacturing regions, while the GHG emissions from running health data centers have global climate impacts.

2.8.2 Estimates of the Carbon Footprint of the Digital Health Sector

Energy use and GHG emissions are the most researched aspects of the digital health sector's environmental footprint. While specific data for health care is limited, we can draw insights from broader ICT sector studies and apply them to the health care context.

The energy use of medical devices, health data centers, and health care networks is a significant contributor to the sector's environmental impact. In the broader ICT context, these components account for approximately 6 to 12 percent of global electricity use. When applied to health care, this suggests that digital health technologies are likely responsible for a substantial portion of the health care sector's energy consumption.

Studies assessing total GHG emissions of digital health have produced varying results, reflecting the challenges in measurement and scope definition. Estimates for the health care sector's overall emissions (including digital and non-digital components) range from 4.4 to 5 percent of global emissions. The digital health component of this is growing but not yet precisely quantified.

These differences become more pronounced in longer-term projections. For example, some studies project that the health care sector's emissions could rise to 6 percent of the global total by 2050 if no mitigating actions are taken. The digital health component of this increase could be substantial, given the rapid adoption of new technologies.

It's important to note that many of these projections rely on extrapolations that may not account for rapid technological changes or efficiency improvements. For instance, early estimates of telemedicine's carbon footprint have been significantly revised as the technology has become more efficient and widespread.

In the case of energy use and associated GHG emissions in digital health:

1. Production phase: This is particularly important for medical devices, especially for battery-powered devices like portable ultrasound machines or wearable health monitors. Studies of consumer electronics suggest that up to 80 percent of a device's lifecycle GHG impact can come from the production phase. This is likely similar to many medical devices.
2. Use phase: For health data centers and networks, the use phase dominates the GHG impact due to their high-energy intensity and constant operation. This includes the energy needed to run electronic health record systems, process medical imaging data, and power AI-driven diagnostic tools.
3. End-of-life phase. While often overlooked, the disposal and recycling of medical electronic waste contribute to the overall carbon footprint.

The relative importance of each phase varies depending on the specific digital health technology.

For example:

- Telemedicine systems: While they reduce travel-related emissions, their use phase (running video consultations, data transmission, etc.) contributes significantly to their carbon footprint.
- AI diagnostic tools: These have a substantial use-phase footprint due to the computational power required, as well as a significant production-phase impact from the hardware needed.
- Electronic health records: The use phase dominates here, with constant data storage and retrieval needs.

It's crucial to note that while digital health technologies contribute to health care's carbon footprint, they also have the potential to reduce emissions in other areas of health care delivery. For example, by optimizing patient flows, reducing unnecessary treatments, and enabling remote care, these technologies could help lower the overall environmental impact of health care.

As the digital health sector continues to evolve rapidly, more research is needed to accurately quantify its specific environmental impact and to develop strategies for minimizing this impact while maximizing health benefits.

2.8.3 Environmental Footprint Beyond Emissions and Energy

While energy use and GHG emissions are the most researched aspects of digital health's environmental footprint, other important impacts include the following:

- Raw material depletion: Production of medical devices and health IT infrastructure requires significant resources, including rare earth minerals.
- Water consumption and quality: Both apply in manufacturing processes and for cooling health data centers.
- Local air quality: This is particularly relevant in regions where medical devices are manufactured.
- Biodiversity: Mining for raw materials and e-waste disposal can significantly impact local ecosystems.
- E-waste generation: The rapid obsolescence of medical devices and health IT equipment contributes to growing electronic waste.

It's crucial to recognize that adverse impacts associated with medical device production and e-waste generation often affect regions far from where these technologies are predominantly used. While developed countries are the primary users of many digital health technologies, considerable environmental harm may accrue in regions that currently benefit less from these advancements.

2.8.4 Digital Health and Health Equity: Environmental Justice Considerations

The distribution of digital health's environmental impact is linked to countries' geographical location and socioeconomic status. This intersection highlights several key points:

- Digital divide in health care: Despite advances in health IT infrastructure, disparities in access and use persist, particularly between high-income and low-income countries.
- Resource extraction: Developing regions are often primary providers of raw materials required for digital health technologies, with extractive processes that can lead to land degradation.
- E-waste destination: Developing countries are often the destination for a significant share of e-waste from global digital health technologies.
- Climate vulnerability: Low-income countries are generally more affected by climate change, which directly impacts their health care systems and options for health-related socioeconomic development.
- Technology access: Low-income countries are less able to afford and harness digital health tools to mitigate various environmental and health impacts.

These factors underscore the need for developed countries and digitally advanced health care systems to assume particular responsibility for ensuring a transition toward a more environmentally sustainable digital health economy that can globally generate inclusive health benefits. Simultaneously, efforts are needed to strengthen the ability of many developing countries to better harness opportunities from digital health in an environmentally sustainable manner, ensuring that the pursuit of advanced health care doesn't come at the cost of environmental degradation in resource-extraction regions.

2.9 Navigating the Intersection of Digital Health and Environmental Sustainability

This chapter has underscored the critical need to give more attention to the interlinkages between the rapidly evolving digital health landscape and environmental sustainability, and their implications for global health equity and development. The expanding scale and changing nature of digital health technologies have environmental implications at all stages of their life cycle—from production to use and disposal. Different countries and health care systems will encounter varying opportunities and challenges at each stage, necessitating a nuanced understanding of how various levels of health care development are affected and how this impacts global health dynamics.

The relationship between digital health and sustainability is bidirectional. Against a backdrop of multiple environmental and health crises and the importance of leveraging digital solutions to improve health care delivery and tackle these challenges, it is increasingly crucial to consider how to reduce the environmental footprint of digital health. However, this presents a double bind for developing countries, particularly those with less advanced health care systems. On one hand, they are often the most vulnerable to potential negative environmental and social effects arising from digital health, relating to raw material extraction for medical devices, carbon emissions from health data centers, and e-waste from obsolete medical equipment. On the other hand, they are less equipped to harness digital health technologies to mitigate risks from climate change and other environmental crises that impact public health.

The transformation of health care through digitalization is an integral part of the significant global changes underway. This is underscored by the urgent need to improve health outcomes, reduce carbon emissions in health care, address widening health inequalities, and enable health care system transformation. In the context of the interrelated nature of Sustainable Development Goals, this requires policy integration and coherence at national, regional, and international levels within the health care sector and beyond.

Against this background, this book seeks to contribute to a better understanding of the environmental impact of the production, use, and end-of-life phases of digital health technologies and infrastructure. The aim is to inform policy debates on digital health, global health equity, and environmentally sustainable and inclusive health care development.

While digital health tools and solutions can be used to reduce the global environmental impact of health care and bring health-related Sustainable Development Goals back on track, positive outcomes cannot be taken for granted. As shown in this chapter, the overall environmental footprint of digital health is hard to assess and remains largely unknown. Identifying opportunities and risks from digital health is hampered by a lack of agreement on what constitutes the digital health sector, what criteria to include in environmental impact assessments of health care technologies, a lack of broadly agreed-upon methodologies to measure impact, and a scarcity of data specific to health care contexts.

The remainder of this book will explore the direct environmental impacts along the three main stages of the digital health technology life cycle. We will focus on the environmental impacts of the production phase of medical devices and health IT infrastructure, the use phase with special attention to health data centers and emerging AI applications in health care, and the end-of-life phase with the potential for fostering more circularity in digital health. We will also explore indirect and rebound effects from digital health use, such as in telemedicine. Finally, we will discuss actions and policies to facilitate a more environmentally sustainable digital health sector that is conducive to inclusive global health development.

By thoroughly examining these aspects, we aim to provide health care leaders, policymakers, and innovators with the insights needed to build a digital health future that not only improves health outcomes but also safeguards the health of our planet. The path forward requires balancing the immense potential of digital health with careful consideration of its environmental impact, ensuring that our efforts to heal do not inadvertently harm the environment upon which all health ultimately depends.

Chapter 3

Digital Health Trends and Their Material Footprint

3.1 The Expanding Material Footprint of Digital Health

The digital transformation of health care, while promising significant improvements in patient care and health outcomes, brings with it a considerable material footprint. This chapter explores the complex relationship between advancing digital health technologies and their environmental impact, with a particular focus on the production phase of the digital health life cycle.

The production of digital health technologies, encompassing everything from wearable health monitors to advanced imaging equipment and health IT infrastructure, marks the beginning of their life cycle. This phase, which includes raw material extraction, refining, component production, and manufacturing, accounts for a significant portion of digital health's overall environmental footprint.

Contrary to initial expectations, the digitalization of health care has not led to dematerialization. Instead, the global material footprint for health care technologies has grown substantially, raising urgent sustainability concerns. The International Resource Panel warns that without concerted action, material resource extraction could increase by almost 60 percent between 2020 and 2060, far exceeding what's required to meet essential health needs aligned with the Sustainable Development Goals.

This material footprint is highly unequal across the globe. High-income countries, with their advanced health care systems, have a significantly larger per capita material footprint for health care technologies compared to lower-income countries. This disparity reflects broader inequalities in health care access and technology adoption, highlighting the need for more equitable approaches to digital health implementation.

The environmental implications of this growing material demand are profound. Resource extraction and processing for health care technologies contribute significantly to climate change, biodiversity loss, and pollution—the triple planetary crisis. As demand surges for materials used in digital health devices and infrastructure, concerns about resource depletion and environmental degradation intensify.

Against this backdrop, this chapter aims to provide a comprehensive examination of the material footprint of digital health, with emphasis on the following key areas:

- the increasing material demands of digital health technologies, from AI-powered diagnostic tools to telemedicine infrastructure
- the environmental impact of extracting and processing materials for health IT infrastructure, including rare earth elements used in medical imaging equipment
- demand projections and supply responses related to transition minerals crucial for digital health technologies
- the geopolitical dynamics of international minerals markets as they relate to health care technology production
- opportunities for developing countries to participate more equitably in the digital health supply chain, moving beyond raw material provision to higher-value production

- the environmental and social implications of mining for health care technology materials, including human rights considerations
- strategies for minimizing the environmental footprint of digital health device production while maximizing health benefits and economic opportunities
- the need for sustainable and ethical sourcing practices in the medical technology industry
- exploring circular economy principles in medical device manufacturing to reduce waste and resource consumption

By examining these aspects, we aim to provide health care leaders, policymakers, and innovators with crucial insights into the material implications of digital health trends. This knowledge is essential for developing strategies that can harness the benefits of digital health technologies while minimizing their environmental impact and promoting more equitable global health development.

The chapter emphasizes the need to consider the shift to digital health as part of a broader transition to sustainable health care. This transition requires vast amounts of minerals and metals, highlighting the interconnectedness of digital innovation and resource management. As we navigate this complex landscape, balancing the immense potential of digital health with careful consideration of its environmental impact becomes paramount.

Our analysis will use the term "transition minerals and metals" to refer to the resources crucial for this shift toward digital and sustainable health care. By thoroughly examining the production phase of digital health technologies, we can better understand the challenges and opportunities that lie ahead in building a health care future that is both technologically advanced and environmentally responsible.

The notion that digitalization in health care would lead to dematerialization by moving activities from the physical to the virtual realm has not been borne out in reality. While digital health is often associated with intangible concepts like "virtual care" or "cloud-based health records," the underlying infrastructure is far from immaterial. In fact, digital health is relatively material intensive, involving significant physical resources, particularly in the production of medical devices and health IT infrastructure, not to mention its high energy demands during use.

Estimations of materials used specifically for digital health are scarce, but we can draw insights from broader digitalization trends. This section discusses the material composition of digital health devices and infrastructure, focusing on minerals and metals, and presents trends leading to increased demand for resources also needed for low-carbon technologies.

3.2 Material Composition of Digital Health Hardware and Infrastructure

Digital health relies heavily on physical components, consuming large amounts of materials to produce medical devices, including batteries powering portable equipment, and to build health IT infrastructure such as hospital networks and health data centers.

While health data itself is intangible, it requires physical support systems:

- patient-facing devices: wearable health monitors, smart medical devices, tablets for telehealth
- health care provider equipment: advanced imaging machines, AI-powered diagnostic tools, telemedicine systems
- data transmission infrastructure: hospital networks, secure health data transmission systems
- data storage: health data centers for electronic health records and AI processing

These digital health technologies are composed of plastics, glass, ceramics, and numerous minerals and metals. For instance, a typical medical tablet might contain over sixty elements from the periodic table, a significant increase from simpler medical devices of the past.

The high intensity of minerals and metals in digital health implies a shift from dependence on traditional medical supplies to reliance on multiple elements in the periodic table. Many of these materials are considered "critical minerals," holding significance for both digital health and low-carbon technologies.

Digital health devices often require these materials in tiny amounts and high purity, complicating recycling efforts. Moreover, the high levels of purity needed are ensured through energy-intensive processing. Declining mineral concentration in ores means huge amounts must be extracted to derive the final mineral content needed for medical devices.

While minerals and metals are essential for digital health even in small quantities, their influence on global markets varies. For some, their application in health care represents a relatively small share of global demand, while for others, medical technology is a major consumer.

Key materials in digital health include aluminum, cobalt, copper, gold, lithium, rare earth elements, and silicon. These elements are crucial for various aspects of digital health technologies, from the conductivity of medical sensors to the energy storage in portable medical devices.

As digital health continues to evolve, the demand for these materials is likely to increase, both in volume and in variety. This trend raises important questions about resource sustainability, supply chain resilience, and the environmental impact of advancing health care technologies. Balancing the benefits of digital health innovations with responsible resource management will be a key challenge for the health care sector moving forward.

3.3 Digital Health Trends Contributing to Increased Demand for Minerals and Metals

The rapid digitalization of health care cannot occur without the significant use of physical raw materials, including minerals and metals. Several factors influence the increasing global demand for these materials in health care, such as population aging, rising chronic disease prevalence, and the push for more advanced medical technologies.

While the recent surge in mineral demand is often attributed to low-carbon technologies, the exponential growth in digital health devices and infrastructure further accentuates the need for increased extraction of minerals and metals. This section provides evidence of evolving trends in digital health that are driving this demand.

Dynamics of increased material consumption and digitalization trends

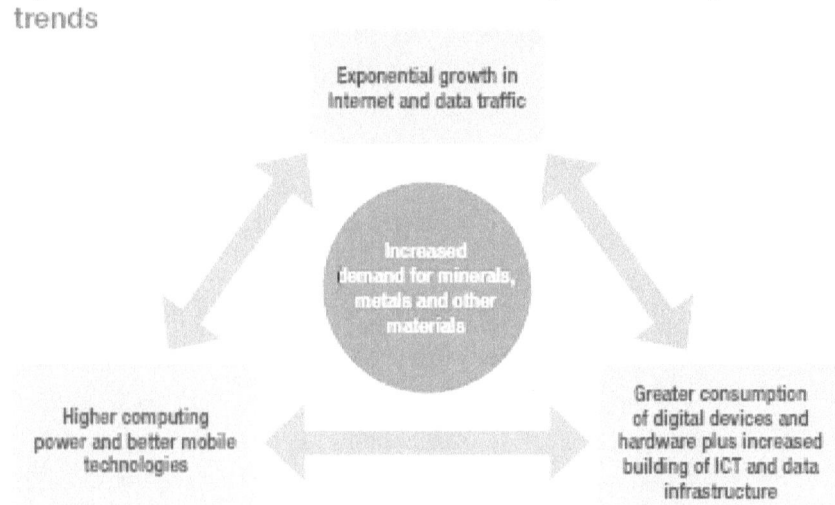

e: UNCTAD

1. Health Data Traffic and Processing

- Global health data volume is growing exponentially. It's estimated that health care data will grow at a compound annual growth rate of over 30 percent through 2025, reaching 2,314 exabytes.
- Telemedicine and remote patient monitoring are major contributors to increased health data traffic. Video consultations, in particular, consume significant bandwidth.

- AI in health care, including imaging analysis and predictive modeling, requires processing vast amounts of data, driving demand for advanced computing infrastructure.

2. Digital Health Devices and Hardware

- Wearable health devices: Global shipments of wearable health monitors are projected to grow from about 520 million units in 2023 to 625 million by 2027.
- Smart medical devices: The Internet of Medical Things is expanding rapidly, with an estimated 20–30 billion connected medical devices expected by 2025.
- Medical imaging equipment: Advanced imaging technologies (MRI, CT, PET scanners) continue to evolve, requiring more sophisticated components.

3. Health IT Infrastructure

- Hospital networks: Upgrading to 5G and Wi-Fi 6 to support increased data loads from connected medical devices and telemedicine.
- Health data centers: Growing demand for storage and processing power to handle electronic health records, AI applications, and big data analytics in health care.

4. Emerging Technologies in Health Care

- AI and machine learning: Increasing adoption for diagnostics, drug discovery, and personalized medicine requires significant computational resources.
- 3D printing in health care: Growing use for prosthetics, dental implants, and even tissue engineering, using various metals and polymers.
- Robotics in surgery: Expansion of robotic-assisted surgery systems, which incorporate advanced materials and electronics.

5. Regional Disparities

- High-income countries continue to lead in the adoption of advanced digital health technologies, but rapid growth is expected in emerging markets, particularly in mobile health applications.
- The digital health divide remains significant, with low-income countries having limited access to many advanced medical technologies.

Future Outlook

- The shift to more personalized, predictive, and preventive health care enabled by digital technologies is likely to further increase demand for specialized materials and components.
- Growing emphasis on sustainable health care may drive innovation in material use and recycling within the medical technology sector.

This digital health revolution, while promising significant improvements in patient care and health outcomes, is contributing to increased demand for various minerals and metals. The health care sector must balance the benefits of these technological advancements with considerations of resource sustainability and environmental impact.

3.4 Demand Projections and Supply Responses for Digital Health Minerals

Demand Projections

Assessing future demand for minerals in digital health involves exploring potential scenarios for health care technology development in the coming decades. Until recently, most forecasts did not thoroughly consider the implications of mineral consumption stemming from digital health technologies. However, growing concerns about high mineral demand for both low-carbon and digital technologies have led to more comprehensive analyses.

Two key factors drive mineral demand in digital health:

1.) Expansion of digital health technologies
2.) Overlap with minerals needed for low-carbon technologies

Projections:

- Significant increase in overall mineral demand, regardless of specific health care technology pathways.
- Potential 300 to 500 percent increase in demand for certain minerals (e.g., lithium, cobalt, rare earth elements) by 2050 for combined low-carbon and digital technologies.
- Digital health could account for 15 to 25 percent of the demand for certain critical minerals by 2040.

Specific digital health drivers

- Wearable health devices: 20 to 30 percent annual growth in mineral demand
- Advanced medical imaging: Up to 50 percent increase in rare earth element demand by 2030
- Health data centers: 40 to 60 percent growth in mineral needs for computing and storage infrastructure

Regional variations

- Developed countries and China currently account for most digital health-related mineral consumption
- Rapid growth expected in emerging markets as digital health adoption increases

Challenges in projections

- Variations based on different technology deployment scenarios
- Uncertainty about future resource intensity and recycling rates
- Potential underestimation of demand from conventional health care uses

Supply Responses

To meet the growing mineral demand for digital health technologies, several supply responses are being considered:

a) Increased mining production

- Expansion of existing mines
- Exploration and development of new mineral deposits
- Concerns about environmental and social impacts of increased mining

b) Improved mineral processing

- Development of more efficient extraction and refining technologies
- Focus on reducing waste and environmental footprint

c) Recycling and circular economy

- Increased efforts to recycle minerals from obsolete medical devices
- Design for recyclability in new digital health products
- Potential for 15 to 20 percent of mineral supply from recycling by 2040

d) Alternative materials

- Research into substitute materials for critical minerals
- Development of new alloys or compounds with similar properties

e) Supply chain diversification

- Efforts to reduce reliance on single sources for critical minerals
- Development of new mining projects in diverse geographic locations

f) Stockpiling

- Some countries and companies building strategic reserves of critical minerals

Challenges

- Long lead times for new mining projects (often ten to fifteen years)
- Geopolitical tensions affecting mineral supply chains
- Balancing environmental concerns with increased production
- Need for significant investment in recycling infrastructure
- Technological hurdles in developing viable alternatives

The health care sector must carefully consider these mineral supply-and-demand dynamics to ensure the sustainable growth of digital health technologies. Collaboration between the health care industry, technology companies, and the mining sector will be crucial to addressing these challenges and securing a stable supply of critical minerals for future digital health innovations.

3.5 Supply Responses for Digital Health Minerals in a Resource-Constrained World

The global response to the surging demand for minerals critical to digital health technologies primarily centers on increasing mineral extraction. However, this approach faces significant challenges given the finite nature of Earth's resources.

Current Supply Strategies

a) Increased mining

- Expansion of existing mines and exploration of new deposits
- Growing interest in untapped regions, including deep-sea and space mining
- Increased exploration budgets, with a significant focus on developing countries

b) Investment in critical minerals

- Sharp rise in investment for critical mineral development

- Uncertainty about whether investment will meet rapidly growing demand

c) Supply chain diversification

- Efforts to reduce reliance on single sources for critical minerals
- Development of new mining projects in diverse geographic locations

Challenges and Limitations

a) Time lags

- Several years between investment in exploration and actual mineral production
- Potential short- to medium-term supply deficits

b) Finite resources

- Growing concern about the long-term availability of minerals for digital health and other technologies
- Increasing extraction difficulties and costs as easily accessible deposits are depleted

c) Environmental and social impacts

- Expansion of mining activities raising significant environmental concerns
- Potential for negative social impacts on local communities

d) Intergenerational equity

- Risk of depleting resources needed by future generations
- Potential for creating intergenerational inequality in access to health care technologies

Rethinking Resource Use in Digital Health

a) Circular economy approaches

- Increased focus on recycling and reuse of minerals from obsolete medical devices
- Design for recyclability in new digital health products

b) Material efficiency

- Development of technologies that use critical minerals more efficiently
- Research into alternative materials with similar properties

c) Sustainable design

- Creating digital health technologies with longer lifespans to reduce replacement frequency
- Modular designs that allow for easier upgrades and repairs

d) Prioritization of critical applications

- Focusing the use of scarce minerals on the most essential digital health technologies
- Exploring low-tech alternatives where appropriate

Balancing Innovation and Sustainability

a) Comprehensive impact assessments

- Considering long-term environmental and social impacts of mineral extraction for digital health
- Evaluating the net benefit of digital health technologies against resource use

b) International cooperation

- Developing global standards for sustainable mineral extraction and use in health care
- Sharing technologies and best practices for efficient resource use

c) Investment in research

- Exploring novel materials and technologies that reduce reliance on scarce minerals
- Developing more efficient mineral processing and recycling technologies

The digital health sector must navigate the complex challenge of advancing health care technologies while respecting the limits of a finite planet. This requires a paradigm shift from a linear "extract, use, discard" model to a circular, resource-efficient approach. Balancing the immense potential of digital health innovations with responsible resource management will be crucial for ensuring sustainable and equitable health care advancements for current and future generations.

The global electronics production chain

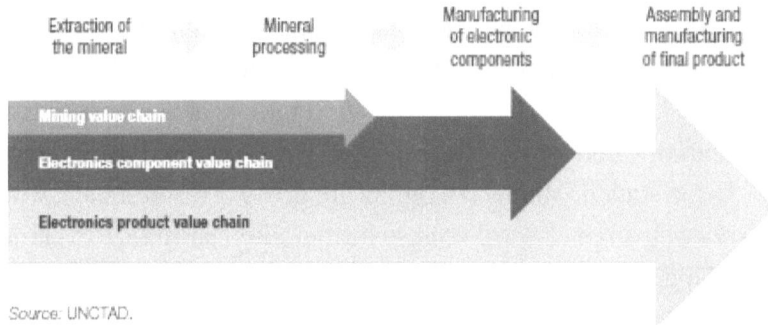

Source: UNCTAD.

3.6 Impacts of the Production Phase on the Planet and People

The production of digital health devices and health care IT infrastructure requires intensive use of minerals and metals, making this lifecycle phase responsible for significant environmental and social impacts associated with mining. As we embrace AI and digital technologies in health care, it's crucial to understand and address these impacts to truly uphold our principle of "First, do no harm."

The following are among the key environmental and social impacts:

1. GHG emissions and energy use: Mining for materials used in medical devices and health IT infrastructure is energy intensive and often relies on fossil fuels. This contributes significantly to global GHG emissions, potentially offsetting some of the environmental benefits of digital health technologies.
2. Water use and pollution: Extraction and processing of minerals for health care technologies require vast amounts of water, often in water-stressed areas. This can lead to water scarcity for local populations and wildlife. Additionally, mining operations can contaminate water sources with toxic chemicals, impacting both human and environmental health.
3. Ecosystem and biodiversity loss: Mining for health care technology materials can threaten vulnerable ecosystems, particularly when it occurs in areas of high biodiversity. This loss of biodiversity could ironically undermine future medical discoveries and public health.
4. Deforestation: Mining is a significant driver of deforestation, which not only impacts local ecosystems but also contributes to climate change, potentially exacerbating global health challenges.
5. Community displacement: Mining activities can lead to displacement of communities, particularly indigenous peoples, disrupting livelihoods and cultural ties to the land. This raises serious ethical questions about the cost of health care advancement.

6. Occupational health and safety: Mining often involves hazardous working conditions, with risks of injuries, illnesses, and long-term health impacts. Ironically, the production of health technologies may be compromising the health of workers in the supply chain.
7. Child labor and human rights violations: In some regions, mining for materials used in health care technologies involves child labor and other human rights abuses. This presents a stark ethical dilemma for the health care sector.
8. Inequality and gender issues: Mining operations can exacerbate local inequalities, particularly affecting women and marginalized communities.

These impacts are often more severe in developing countries and least developed countries (LDCs), which may have limited capabilities to address the negative externalities of mining. As the demand for digital health technologies grows, these impacts could potentially double, or even quadruple, by 2060 if not properly addressed.

It's important to note that these environmental and social impacts are interconnected. Environmental degradation from mining often leads to social impacts and human rights violations. For instance, water pollution from mining can lead to health issues in local communities, infringing on their right to health and clean water.

As we advance digital health technologies, we must consider the entire lifecycle of these innovations. The health care sector has a responsibility to ensure that our efforts to improve health outcomes do not come at the cost of environmental degradation and human rights violations in mining communities.

Addressing these challenges will require concerted efforts from health care providers, technology companies, policymakers, and mining operators.

The following are among the potential strategies:

1. Investing in renewable energy for mining operations
2. Implementing strict environmental and social standards in the health care technology supply chain
3. Supporting research into alternative, more sustainable materials for medical devices
4. Promoting circular economy principles in health care technology design and disposal
5. Engaging with local communities and respecting indigenous rights in mining areas
6. Improving transparency and traceability in the health care technology supply chain

By tackling these issues head-on, we can work toward a truly sustainable and ethical digital health future—one that improves human health without compromising the health of our planet or the well-being of vulnerable communities. This holistic approach to "First, do no harm" is essential for the long-term sustainability and credibility of digital health innovations.

3.7 Conclusions

This chapter has examined the production phase of digital health technologies, with a focus on the mining and processing of minerals essential for these innovations. It has revealed that the digital transformation of health care is a material-intensive process, raising significant environmental and ethical concerns.

The health care sector is undergoing a profound transformation, driven by AI and digital technologies that are highly dependent on minerals and metals. Without these materials, the digitalization of health care would not be possible. The demand for these resources reflects the rapid development of new medical technologies, which necessitates an increasing number of devices and the continuous expansion of digital health infrastructure.

This surge in demand for minerals raises major geopolitical and developmental challenges. In the wake of global supply chain disruptions, some reorganization of production is occurring. Developed countries importing these minerals and manufacturing medical devices are seeking to secure supplies, including through increased domestic production and new international alliances. This shift in focus from economic efficiency to security has implications for global health equity and environmental sustainability.

For developing countries, this scenario could provide opportunities for economic development, provided they can add more value to their mineral resources. However, it's crucial to address the potential environmental and social impacts of mining and manufacturing in these countries, including human rights concerns.

From a global perspective, there is a risk of overmining and manufacturing overcapacity in the health care technology sector. This could lead to a waste of resources that could have been used for other developmental purposes, including direct health care provision.

Addressing the growing demand for minerals in health care technology will require rethinking our models of consumption and production. This includes not only increasing the primary supply from mines and secondary supply from recycling but also reducing excessive consumption where possible. Given the significant digital health divides between developed and developing countries, there may be more margin for consumption reduction in developed health care systems.

Technological advances offer some hope, potentially leading to increased resource efficiency or mineral substitutes in medical devices. For example, changes in battery chemistry for portable medical equipment may reduce the use of certain minerals. Recycling medical electronic waste is also a crucial strategy to reduce mineral extraction.

Moving forward, the health care sector must adopt a more balanced, comprehensive approach that considers both supply and demand aspects. This approach should combine the interests of developing and developed countries, exporters and importers, while aiming for more responsible and sustainable consumption and production in health care technology.

Such an approach will require changes in how we develop, produce, and use digital health technologies to make them more environmentally sustainable and socially responsible. This transformation should be enabled, promoted, and regulated by public policies, including regional and global governance structures specific to health care technology.

As we continue to explore the lifecycle of digital health technologies in the following chapters, we must keep in mind that truly adhering to the principle of "First, do no harm" extends beyond individual patient care to encompass the global impacts of our health care practices. By addressing these challenges, we can work toward a digital health future that improves human health without compromising the health of our planet or the well-being of vulnerable communities involved in the production of these technologies.

Chapter 4

Environmental Impacts in the Use Phase of Digital Health Technologies

4.1 Introduction

The rapidly expanding adoption of digital health technologies worldwide is transforming health care delivery while simultaneously contributing to the sector's environmental footprint. As we strive to improve patient outcomes and health care efficiency through digitalization, we must also consider the environmental implications of these innovations throughout their life cycle.

This chapter explores the primary environmental impacts stemming from the utilization of digital health devices, health data transmission networks, and health care data centers in light of current trends and developments. The operation of these technologies activates a complex network of physical systems, including various medical devices, health IT infrastructure, servers, cables, and routers, all of which require substantial energy and resources to function.

To comprehensively assess the environmental footprint, we focus on three key areas:

1. Greenhouse gas (GHG) emissions linked to energy use
2. Water stress from cooling systems, particularly in health care data centers
3. Noise pollution from health IT infrastructure

The growing demand for digital health services is generating an ever-increasing need for health data to be transmitted, stored, and processed. This escalation triggers the use of a series of complex physical systems, each with its own environmental impact. As digital technologies become ubiquitous across all areas of health care, it is crucial to thoroughly understand, monitor, and manage these environmental impacts.

While energy consumption and associated GHG emissions in health care IT have drawn growing attention, estimates of the electricity consumption and carbon footprint of digital health technologies vary considerably due to differing methodologies and data sources. Other environmental considerations, such as water consumption by health care data centers, are often overlooked when assessing the use phase's environmental footprint.

The following are among the key areas of focus in this chapter:

- energy consumption of IoMT devices and wearable health monitors
- power requirements for AI-driven diagnostic tools and telemedicine platforms
- environmental impact of storing and processing vast amounts of health data
- water usage in cooling health care data centers
- GHG emissions associated with the operation of digital health infrastructure

Improving the evidence base in this context is vital to enhance public understanding, inform health care policymaking, and influence behavior among health care providers, technology companies, and patients to achieve environmentally sustainable digital health practices.

The aims of this chapter are as follows:

1. Summarize the current state of research on the environmental impacts of digital health technologies in use
2. Identify key data gaps and uncertainties specific to the health care sector
3. Outline potential future trends in digital health and their environmental implications
4. Explore opportunities for mitigating various environmental risks to enhance the sustainability of digital health

The chapter is structured as follows:

- Section 1 provides an overview of environmental impacts arising from the operation of health care data centers, health data transmission networks, and digital health devices.
- Section 2 takes a deep dive into health care data centers, focusing on their impacts at both global and local levels.
- Section 3 investigates how potential environmental impacts depend on specific digital health services and underlying technologies, including emerging innovations such as AI in diagnostics, blockchain for health records, 5G-enabled telemedicine, and the Internet of Medical Things.
- Section 4 provides concluding observations and implications for building a sustainable health care future.

As we examine these impacts, we must constantly balance the immense potential of digital health to improve patient care and health outcomes with our responsibility to minimize harm to the environment. This holistic approach to "First, do no harm" is essential for building a truly sustainable health care future with AI and digital technologies.

By understanding and addressing the environmental impacts in the use phase of digital health technologies, we can work toward a health care system that not only heals patients but also treads lightly on our planet. This knowledge is crucial for health care leaders, policymakers, and innovators committed to harnessing the power of digital health while upholding the principle of "First, do no harm"—not just for individual patients but also for our planet as a whole.

4.2 Main Environmental Impacts of Digital Health Technologies

In terms of energy use and greenhouse gas (GHG) emissions, it is estimated that 56 to 80 percent of the total life cycle impact of digital health technologies can be attributed to the use phase. However, this share varies depending on the specific health care technologies used and the energy mix associated with their operation.

For health care data centers and health data transmission networks, due to their high-energy intensity and continuous operation (24/7), the use phase may account for over 80 percent of GHG emissions over their life cycle. In contrast, for connected medical devices, the use phase represents less than half of the life cycle energy and GHG impact. For battery-powered medical devices—such as portable health monitors and tablets used in clinical settings—the share is even lower, typically around 10 to 20 percent. Approximately 80 percent of the life cycle energy and GHG impact of a medical tablet or smartphone used in health care comes from the manufacturing stage.

Greenhouse gas emissions

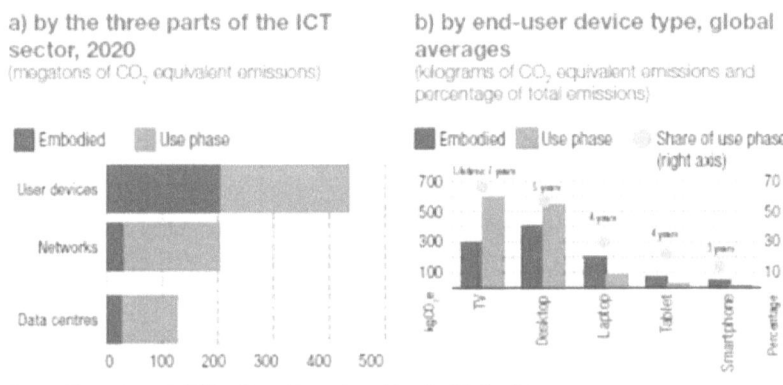

a) by the three parts of the ICT sector, 2020
(megatons of CO_2 equivalent emissions)

b) by end-user device type, global averages
(kilograms of CO_2 equivalent emissions and percentage of total emissions)

Source: Malmodin et al. (2024, left) and Malmodin and Lundén (2018, right).
Notes: Carbon emissions for device types (right) are representative of global averages. Actual carbon emissions

According to recent estimates, the digital health sector uses about 3 to 5 percent of global electricity in the use stage and accounts for about 1 to 2 percent of global GHG emissions. Both electricity consumption and GHG emissions in the use phase have increased in recent years, reflecting the enhanced uptake of various digital health technologies, devices, and services.

Water consumption associated with the use of digital health technologies has received relatively little attention until recently. However, several studies have now stressed that the water footprint is an indispensable part of the overall environmental impact of digital health technologies. This is particularly relevant for health care data centers, which require significant amounts of water for cooling. However, the evidence base is still limited, especially in developing countries. This reflects various factors, including the reluctance of health technology companies to share data and the lack of requirements and incentives for them to do so.

The environmental impacts can be categorized by three main components of digital health infrastructure:

1. End-user devices (e.g., medical tablets, wearable health monitors)

   - primary impact: energy consumption and associated GHG emissions
   - secondary impact: e-waste generation at end of life

2. Health data transmission networks

   - primary impact: energy consumption and associated GHG emissions
   - secondary impact: potential electromagnetic radiation effects

3. Health care data centers

   - primary impacts: (a) energy consumption and associated GHG emissions (b) water consumption for cooling
   - secondary impacts: (a) land use (b) noise pollution

For user devices and networks, energy consumption and the associated GHG emissions are the main environmental impacts under discussion. For health care data centers, water consumption is also a significant concern, particularly in water-stressed regions.

As the digital health sector continues to grow, it's crucial to develop more comprehensive and standardized methods for assessing these environmental impacts. This will enable health care providers, policymakers, and technology companies to make informed decisions that balance the benefits of digital health technologies with their environmental costs, truly embodying the principle of "First, do no harm" on both individual and global scales.

4.2.1. End-User Devices in Digital Health

During the use phase of digital health technologies, end-user devices account for a significant share of GHG emissions. However, this share differs considerably between device types used in health care settings.

For mains-powered medical devices, such as stationary patient monitors or medical imaging equipment, the relatively high level of power consumption means that more than half of life-cycle energy use and emissions can be attributed to the use phase. In contrast, for more energy-efficient devices like medical tablets or wearable health monitors, the production phase is the dominant source of emissions. The greater the number of digital health devices deployed globally, the greater the environmental impact in both the production phase and waste generation at the end of life.

Although the total number of digital health devices has increased rapidly over the past decade, overall energy consumption associated with their use has been found to be relatively stable. This reflects several factors:

1. Shift toward smaller, more energy-efficient devices (e.g., from stationary medical workstations to medical tablets and smartphones)
2. Transition to more energy-efficient screens in medical settings (e.g., from CRT to LCD to more efficient LED screens)
3. Integration of multiple functions into single devices (e.g., smartphones replacing separate medical calculators, reference books, and communication devices)

However, it's important to note that the growing demand for larger screens in medical imaging and telemedicine is offsetting some of the efficiency gains from shifting to more efficient display technologies.

Variations in time frame, scope, assumptions, and data sources result in different estimates of energy use by digital health devices.

For example:

- Medical tablets and smartphones used in health care settings are estimated to consume about 50 TWh to 100 TWh annually.
- Medical IoT devices (such as connected patient monitors and smart medical equipment) may consume an additional 20 TWh to 40 TWh.
- Larger medical equipment (e.g., MRI machines and CT scanners) can contribute significantly to energy consumption, with estimates ranging from 100–200 TWh annually.

Together, these digital health devices may account for 170TWh to 340 TWh of energy consumption annually, equivalent to approximately 0.7 to 1.4 percent of global electricity use. However, it's crucial to note that these figures are estimates and may vary depending on the specific technologies included and the methodologies used.

Typical daily power consumption of computing devices and monitors (watts)

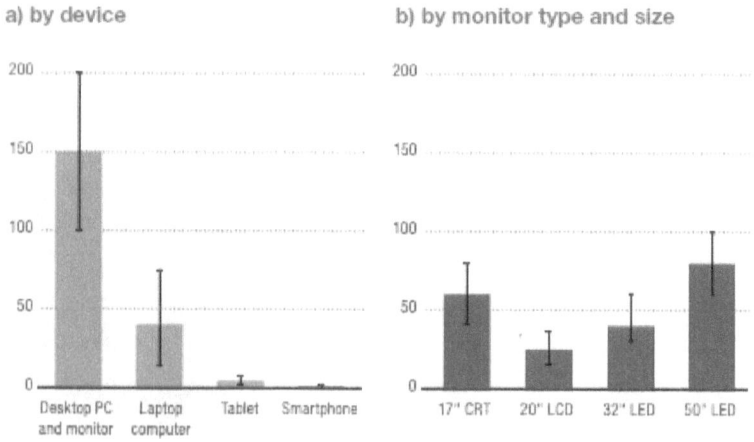

Source: UNCTAD, based on Urban et al. (2017) and Kamiya (2020a).

As the digital health sector continues to evolve, several trends are likely to impact the environmental footprint of end-user devices:

1. Increasing adoption of wearable health monitors and home health devices may lead to a larger number of devices in use, potentially increasing overall energy consumption.
2. Advancements in energy-efficient technologies may help offset the increased number of devices.
3. The shift toward cloud-based health services may reduce the processing power required in end-user devices, potentially decreasing their energy consumption.
4. The growing use of AI in medical devices may increase the computational demands and energy consumption of some devices.

Understanding these trends and their environmental implications is crucial for health care providers, technology developers, and policymakers as they work to balance the benefits of digital health technologies with their environmental impact. This balance is essential to truly uphold the principle of "First, do no harm" in the digital age of health care.

4.2.2 Data Transmission Networks in Health Care

In the context of digital health, data transmission networks play a crucial role in connecting various elements of the health care ecosystem. These networks encompass hospital and clinic networks, telemedicine infrastructure, health information exchanges, and mobile health applications. They are responsible for transmitting vast amounts of sensitive health data between health care providers, patients, and various digital health devices.

Energy Consumption and Efficiency

Health care data transmission networks are estimated to consume a significant amount of energy, contributing to the sector's overall environmental footprint. While exact figures for health care–specific networks are not available, we can draw insights from broader ICT network data:

- Data transmission networks in general consumed an estimated 260 TWh to 360 TWh in 2022, equivalent to 1.1 to 1.5 percent of global electricity use.
- Mobile networks, which are increasingly important for telemedicine and remote patient monitoring, account for about two-thirds of this energy consumption.

The good news is that the energy efficiency of data transmission has greatly improved over the past decade:

- The energy needed to transmit 1 gigabyte (GB) of data through fixed-line networks has been halving approximately every two years.
- Mobile network energy efficiency has improved by 10 to 30 percent annually.
- Each new generation of mobile network uses significantly less energy to transmit the same amount of data than its predecessor.

However, these efficiency gains are often offset by the rapid increase in data traffic, particularly in health care:

- The rise of telemedicine, high-resolution medical imaging sharing, and real-time patient monitoring has led to exponential growth in health care data traffic.
- This increased usage can lead to rebound effects, where total energy consumption rises despite improved efficiency.

Challenges in Measuring Energy Efficiency

While energy per unit of data (e.g., kWh/GB) is a commonly used metric for network energy efficiency, it has limitations in the health care context:

- It doesn't adequately capture the energy performance of last-mile access networks, which are crucial for connecting remote patients or rural health care facilities.

- It fails to accurately measure the energy use of specific digital health services, such as real-time surgical video streaming or AI-powered diagnostic tools, which may have different energy profiles.

To truly understand and monitor energy efficiency progress in health care data transmission networks, we need to track these:

1. Total energy use
2. Energy efficiency indicators based on these factors:

    - number of health care connections
    - peak traffic during critical care periods
    - coverage of health care facilities and patients
    - quality of service for time-sensitive medical applications

Environmental and Health Considerations

While improving energy efficiency is crucial, we must also consider other environmental and health aspects of health care data transmission networks:

1. Electromagnetic radiation: The proliferation of wireless networks for health care applications raises concerns about potential long-term health effects, which need further study.
2. Infrastructure footprint: The physical infrastructure required for robust health care networks (e.g., cell towers, data centers) can have local environmental impacts.
3. E-waste: Frequent upgrades to network equipment to meet growing health care data demands contribute to electronic waste.
4. Data security and privacy: While not directly an environmental concern, ensuring the security and privacy of health data transmitted over these networks is crucial for maintaining patient trust in digital health systems.

As we continue to expand and improve data transmission networks for health care, we must balance the immense benefits of connectivity with its environmental costs. This aligns with our overarching principle of "First, do no harm"—not just in patient care but also in our approach to the planet's health.

Future research and policy efforts should focus on the following areas:

1. Developing health care-specific metrics for network energy efficiency
2. Encouraging the adoption of energy-efficient network technologies in health care settings
3. Exploring ways to optimize health care data traffic to reduce unnecessary energy consumption
4. Investigating the potential of edge computing in health care to reduce long-distance data transmission
5. Ensuring that improvements in network efficiency translate into real reductions in overall energy use and emissions in the health care sector

By addressing these challenges, we can work toward a digital health infrastructure that enhances patient care while minimizing its environmental impact.

4.2.3 Health Care Data Centers: A Growing Environmental Concern

Health care data centers are at the heart of the digital health revolution, storing and processing vast volumes of sensitive patient data, supporting telemedicine services, enabling AI-driven diagnostics, and facilitating health information exchanges. These data centers come in various capacities to support a wide range of digital health services, from electronic health records to complex medical imaging analysis.

The demand for these services is rising rapidly in health care, raising critical questions about their impact on energy use, GHG emissions, water consumption, and other environmental concerns. This growth is driven by several factors:

- Increasing adoption of electronic health records
- Expansion of telemedicine services
- Growing use of AI and machine learning in medical research and diagnostics
- Rising demand for real-time health monitoring and data analysis
- Stricter data retention requirements in health care

As the backbone of digital health infrastructure, health care data centers require immense computing capacity and consequently consume large amounts of both energy and water. This significant resource consumption raises important environmental considerations in our pursuit of advanced digital health solutions. But the environmental impact of health care data centers extends beyond energy and water consumption:

- Land use: Large data centers require significant space, potentially leading to habitat disruption.
- E-waste: Regular hardware upgrades contribute to electronic waste.
- Noise pollution: Cooling systems and backup generators can create noise disturbances.
- Heat island effect: In urban areas, the heat generated by data centers can contribute to local temperature increases.

4.2.3.1 Energy Consumption

Based on recent estimates, global data center electricity consumption (excluding cryptocurrency mining) was 240 TWh to 340 TWh in 2022, representing around 1 to 1.5 percent of global electricity use. While health care–specific figures are not available, it is estimated that health care data centers could account for 10 to 15 percent of this total, given the data-intensive nature of modern medicine.

To put this in perspective, the energy consumption of health care data centers alone could be comparable to the annual electricity consumption of a small country. This level of energy use translates to significant greenhouse gas (GHG) emissions. In 2020, the use phase GHG emissions of data centers were estimated at 95 MtCO2e, three times greater than the emissions from their production stage.

Despite improvements in energy efficiency, the strong increase in workloads handled has resulted in energy use by collocation and hyperscale data center operators expanding by 10 to 30 percent each year since 2020. For thirteen of the largest data center operators, company-wide electricity consumption more than doubled between 2018 and 2022.

4.2.3.2 Water Consumption

Water consumption in health care data centers is primarily associated with cooling systems, which are crucial for maintaining optimal operating conditions for the powerful computers processing health data. For large-scale health care data centers, which have massive computing power and generate substantial heat, effective cooling is essential for uninterrupted operation.

It's important to note that water and electricity consumption in health care data centers are interlinked and need to be considered holistically. While some cooling technologies can operate without water, they may instead consume large amounts of electricity, potentially increasing overall energy-related emissions.

4.2.3.4 Energy Efficiency and Cooling Trends

Global data center energy use appears to have grown less than expected over the past decade, considering the strong expansion in demand for data center services. This has mainly been attributed to the following:

- Efficiency improvements in IT hardware and cooling systems
- A shift from inefficient enterprise data centers toward more efficient cloud and hyperscale data centers

Running applications in the cloud requires 60 to 90 percent less energy than using on-premise data centers. However, smaller data centers serving health care providers that are less reliant on cloud services tend to be much less energy efficient.

Data centers need energy to power IT and infrastructure equipment. Globally, the vast majority of IT-related energy in data centers is consumed by servers (80 percent), followed by storage devices (18 percent) and network equipment (3 percent), while most infrastructure-related energy use is related to cooling.

The efficiency of data centers is often measured by power usage effectiveness (PUE). Currently, the global average PUE in data centers is around 1.6, meaning that for every 1.6 kWh of electricity used, 1 kWh is used for IT and 0.6 kWh for cooling and other non-IT equipment.

Given the significant share of cooling in overall energy use by data centers, reducing such energy use has become a major focus for operators. The following are among the strategies that can be considered:

- more efficient cooling systems, including hot and cold aisle-contained cooling systems
- allowing data centers to operate at slightly higher temperatures
- locating data centers in cooler climates
- exploring liquid cooling methods, such as immersion cooling

Innovative approaches are being tested, such as underwater data centers, which have shown promising results in energy efficiency and reduced failure rates. Looking ahead, several factors will influence the energy consumption and efficiency of health care data centers:

- the pace of overall demand growth for data center services, particularly from emerging technologies like AI in health care diagnostics and personalized medicine

- further energy efficiency improvements in IT hardware and cooling technologies
- the extent to which existing workloads in health care enterprise data centers will be migrated to the cloud
- broader trends in digital health technologies that influence data center developments, such as a greater need for low-latency services for remote surgeries

4.3 Implications of Different Digital Health Services and Technologies

Environmental impacts in the use phase of digital health are affected not only by the types of devices used but also by the specific activities and technologies involved. Digital health services encompass a wide variety of applications, from electronic health records (EHRs) and telemedicine, to AI-powered diagnostics and medical imaging analysis. These digital health services differ in how they employ technologies and infrastructure, leading to varying environmental footprints.

This section discusses the environmental impact of some widely used digital health services and emerging technologies:

4.3.1 Telemedicine and Video Consultations

Telemedicine services, particularly video consultations, have seen a significant rise in adoption. The energy and carbon footprint of these services depends on several factors:

- data center processing for video streaming and medical data analysis
- data transmission through networks
- energy consumption of devices used by health care providers and patients

Recent studies have shown that the environmental impact of video consultations is generally lower than previously estimated, especially when compared to the emissions associated with patient travel for in-person visits. However, as telemedicine usage increases, its cumulative environmental impact will need careful monitoring.

4.3.2 Electronic Health Records (EHRs) and Health Information Exchange

EHRs and health information exchange systems require continuous data storage and processing. Their environmental impact is primarily associated with the following:

- energy consumption of data centers hosting health records
- network energy use for data transmission between health care providers
- device energy use for accessing and updating records

While EHRs have significantly reduced paper waste in health care, their digital footprint needs consideration. Optimizing data storage and implementing energy-efficient data management practices can help mitigate this impact.

4.3.3 AI-Powered Diagnostic Tools and Medical Imaging Analysis

Advanced AI applications in health care, such as diagnostic tools and medical imaging analysis, are computationally intensive. Their environmental implications include the following:

- high energy consumption for training and running AI models
- increased data center cooling requirements due to intensive computing
- potential for increased e-waste as health care providers upgrade to AI-compatible hardware

However, these technologies also have the potential to improve diagnostic accuracy and efficiency, potentially reducing the need for repeated tests and their associated environmental impacts.

4.3.4 Internet of Medical Things and Remote Patient Monitoring

The proliferation of connected medical devices and wearable health monitors contributes to the growing Internet of Medical Things. The following are among the environmental considerations:

- energy consumption of numerous small devices
- increased network traffic and associated energy use
- data center energy use for processing and storing continuous streams of health data

While these technologies can improve patient care and potentially reduce hospital visits, their cumulative energy consumption needs careful management.

4.3.5 Blockchain in Health Care

Blockchain technology is being explored for secure health data management and drug traceability. The following are among the environmental implications:

- high energy consumption, particularly for proof-of-work consensus mechanisms
- increased data center cooling requirements due to intensive computing

The health care sector needs to carefully weigh the benefits of blockchain against its potential environmental costs.

4.3.6 5G and Edge Computing in Health Care

The rollout of 5G networks and edge computing has significant implications for digital health:

- potential for reduced latency and improved real-time health monitoring
- increased energy efficiency in data transmission
- shift in energy consumption from centralized data centers to distributed edge computing nodes

While these technologies can enhance health care delivery, their overall environmental impact will depend on implementation strategies and energy sources used.

4.3.7 Virtual Reality and the Metaverse in Health Care

The emergence of the *health care metaverse*—a digital immersive environment for medical communication, training, and treatment—utilizes technologies such as virtual reality (VR) and augmented reality (AR). This digital realm presents both opportunities and challenges for sustainable health care.

Potential Benefits

- Reduced travel emissions: VR and AR can replace physical travel for medical consultations, conferences, and training, potentially reducing associated GHG emissions.
- Enhanced medical training: Immersive technologies allow for realistic medical simulations without the need for physical resources, potentially reducing material waste.
- Remote patient monitoring: AR applications could enable more effective remote patient care, reducing the need for in-person visits.

Environmental Concerns

- Energy-intensive infrastructure: The health care metaverse requires advanced computing power, fast networks, and sophisticated end-user devices, all of which consume substantial amounts of electricity and water.
- Increased data center demand: The need for real-time, high-fidelity rendering in medical applications could significantly increase data-center energy consumption.
- Hardware production and e-waste: The production of VR/AR devices for health care applications contributes to resource depletion and potential e-waste.

While specific estimates for the health care metaverse are not available, general metaverse GHG emissions could reach 115 MtCO2e by 2030, accounting for approximately 0.5 percent of global carbon emissions. The health care sector's portion of this would depend on adoption rates and specific applications.

Some researchers believe that the metaverse, including its health care applications, could potentially reduce more emissions than it causes by:

- accelerating the adoption of telemedicine and remote care
- improving the efficiency of medical training and reducing associated travel
- enabling more precise and efficient health care delivery through AR-guided procedures

As digital health technologies continue to evolve and become more sophisticated, their environmental footprint is likely to grow. Managing and mitigating these impacts will require concerted efforts from health care providers, technology companies, policymakers, and patients.

The following are among the key strategies:

- prioritizing energy efficiency in the development of digital health technologies
- implementing renewable energy sources for powering digital health infrastructure
- optimizing data management practices to reduce unnecessary storage and processing
- considering the full lifecycle environmental impact of digital health technologies, from production to end-of-life
- balancing the benefits of advanced digital health services with their environmental costs

By carefully considering these factors, the health care sector can harness the power of digital technologies to improve patient care while minimizing environmental harm, truly embodying the principle of "First, do no harm" in the digital age.

Here's a rewritten version of the concluding observations and recommendations section, adapted for the book *First, Do No Harm: Building a Sustainable Health Care Future with AI and Digital Technologies*:

4.5 Concluding Observations and Recommendations

This chapter has examined the environmental footprint of digital health technologies during their use phase, with particular attention to health care data centers due to their significant environmental impact. As digital health continues to evolve and expand, the role of these data centers is expected to grow, driven by emerging technologies and increasing digitalization in health care.

Key Observations

1. Holistic environmental assessment: It's crucial not to focus solely on individual environmental indicators (such as GHG emissions) when assessing the sustainability of digital health. A comprehensive approach should prioritize energy efficiency and responsible water consumption in health care IT infrastructure.
2. Uncertainty in long-term forecasts: Given the rapid pace of technological progress in health care and the difficulties in measuring energy use and water consumption, long-term forecasts of the environmental footprint of digital health beyond the next five years are highly uncertain.
3. Energy efficiency limits: If current energy efficiency trends in computing continue, processor efficiency limits could be reached by around 2040, potentially impacting the future energy consumption of digital health technologies.
4. Growing data center energy use: Health care data center energy use is expected to increase significantly due to growing demand from compute-intensive applications like AI-driven diagnostics and the global expansion of digital health services.

Recommendations

1. Renewable energy adoption: Health care organizations should prioritize powering data centers through renewable energy sources to curb GHG emissions while also reducing emissions from supply chains.
2. Water resource management: More attention must be given to mitigating the impact of health care data centers on scarce water resources, particularly in water-stressed regions.
3. Transparency in reporting: Health care technology companies should transparently report data on relevant environmental indicators, including the energy and carbon footprints of AI applications in health care.

4. Government leadership: Governments should accelerate research and development to advance more efficient, next-generation health care technologies and systems. They should also promote improved energy efficiency of health care data centers through regulation and renewable energy mandates.
5. Agile policymaking: Regulations need to provide long-term planning security for private-sector investment in digital health while recognizing the dynamic character of the health care IT sector.
6. Demand response programs: Regulators should ensure that electricity market design provides clear and sufficient price signals for health care data centers to participate in demand-response programs.
7. Infrastructure codevelopment: In developing countries, governments and utilities could consider opportunities to codevelop local electricity and water infrastructure with new health care data center projects, expanding access to these resources in communities.
8. Circularity and sufficiency: Sector regulations are important to foster circularity and sufficiency in health care technology. This could include requirements for modular design in medical devices to facilitate repairs and upgrades.
9. AI impact assessment: Given the growing use of AI in health care, it's crucial to weigh the environmental risks and benefits of using AI for various medical applications. Regulators could consider introducing specific environmental disclosure requirements for AI in health care to enhance transparency across the supply chain.
10. Education and awareness: Health care professionals and patients should be educated about the environmental impact of digital health technologies and encouraged to adopt sustainable practices in their use of these technologies.

By implementing these recommendations, the health care sector can work toward a more sustainable digital future, one that improves patient outcomes while minimizing environmental harm. This approach embodies the principle of "First, do no harm" in its broadest sense, encompassing both individual patient care and global environmental stewardship.

Chapter 5

The End-of-Life Challenge: Managing Digital Health Waste

5.1 Introduction

This chapter focuses on the final stage of the digital health technology life cycle: the end-of-life phase. As we embrace AI and digital technologies to improve health care, we must also confront the growing challenge of electronic waste (e-waste) generated by obsolete medical devices and health IT infrastructure.

The rapid pace of technological advancement in health care, while bringing numerous benefits, has led to an alarming increase in digitalization-related waste. This trend presents both challenges and opportunities from economic and environmental sustainability perspectives. Current waste-management practices in health care are often insufficient, marked by inadequate recycling and informal handling, especially in developing countries. Addressing this situation is crucial to mitigate the environmental and health impacts of improperly disposed digital health devices.

This chapter advocates for a more circular approach to digital health, emphasizing the need to extend the lifespan of medical devices and improve recycling efficiency. Such an approach would not only alleviate pressure on raw material supplies but could also create new economic opportunities within the health care sector.

The following are among the key areas:

1. Global trends in digital health-related waste
2. Environmental and health impacts of improper disposal of medical electronic devices
3. Current waste management practices in health care and their limitations
4. Opportunities for implementing circular economy principles in digital health
5. The role of policy and global coordination in addressing the e-waste challenge in health care

The challenge ahead involves developing coordinated global efforts and robust policies for waste treatment and circularity throughout the lifecycle of digital health technologies. By addressing these issues, we can ensure that our efforts to improve health outcomes through digital innovation do not come at the cost of environmental degradation.

As we explore these topics, we'll consider how the health care sector can uphold the principle of "First, do no harm," not just in patient care but also in its approach to environmental stewardship. This chapter aims to provide health care leaders, policymakers, and technology innovators with insights and strategies to build a more sustainable digital health future—one that heals both people and the planet.

5.2 Defining Digital Health-Related Waste

Defining waste-related to digital health technologies is not straightforward. It falls under the broader category of "electrical and electronic waste" (e-waste), also known as "waste electrical and electronic equipment"

(WEEE). However, digital health waste has unique characteristics and challenges that require specific consideration.

In the context of health care, digital health-related waste encompasses a wide range of items:

1. Medical devices: include outdated or nonfunctional diagnostic equipment, patient monitoring systems, and medical imaging devices.
2. Health care IT infrastructure: includes obsolete servers, network equipment, and data storage devices used in health care facilities
3. Wearable health technologies: include smartwatches, fitness trackers, and other patient-worn devices used for health monitoring.
4. Mobile Health devices: Smartphones, tablets, and other portable devices used for telemedicine or health data collection.
5. Specialized health care equipment: AI-powered diagnostic tools, robotic surgical systems, and other advanced medical technologies.

The challenge in defining digital health waste lies in determining when a device becomes "waste." This can be particularly complex in health care settings where:

- Devices may be decommissioned due to regulatory requirements rather than malfunction.
- Rapid technological advancements may render equipment obsolete before the end of its functional lifespan.
- Some components may be reusable or recyclable, blurring the line between "waste" and valuable resources.

Legal and Statistical Definitions

Legally, the Basel Convention on the Control of Transboundary Movements of Hazardous Wastes and Their Disposal provides a framework for defining e-waste, which includes digital health equipment. Recent amendments have added precision to this definition, particularly regarding hazardous and nonhazardous e-waste.

Statistically, the Global E-Waste Statistics Partnership defines e-waste as discarded electrical and electronic equipment (EEE) and its parts. While this definition encompasses digital health technologies, it doesn't specifically categorize them.

For the purposes of this book, we propose defining digital health-related waste as follows:

Any electrical or electronic equipment used in health care settings for diagnosis, treatment, monitoring, or health data management that has been discarded by the owner as waste without the intention of reuse, including all components, sub-assemblies, and consumables that are part of the product at the time of discarding.

This definition aims to capture the unique aspects of digital health technologies while aligning with broader e-waste definitions.

Challenges in Measurement

Measuring digital health-related waste presents several challenges:

1. Rapid technological evolution: The definition of what constitutes digital health equipment is constantly changing as new technologies emerge.
2. Interconnected devices: Many medical devices are becoming "smart" and interconnected, blurring the line between traditional medical equipment and digital health technologies.
3. Data security: Health care devices often contain sensitive patient data, requiring special handling and disposal procedures.
4. Regulatory compliance: Health care e-waste must often meet stricter disposal standards due to potential biohazards or data privacy concerns.

5. Global disparities: The management of digital health waste varies significantly between developed and developing countries, making global assessments challenging.

As we advance toward a more digitalized health care future, understanding and managing the waste generated by these technologies becomes crucial. The definition and measurement of digital health-related waste must evolve to keep pace with technological advancements and ensure that our efforts to improve health care don't inadvertently harm the environment.

In the following sections, we will explore the current trends in digital health waste generation, its environmental impacts, and its strategies for more sustainable management, always keeping in mind our guiding principle: "First, do no harm."

5.3 Trends in Digital Health-Related Waste

Tracking the entire lifecycle and global trends in digital health-related waste presents significant challenges. Much of this waste, like broader e-waste, is not formally managed, recorded, or documented, often escaping scrutiny or monitoring. This is due to informal sector activities, illegal trade, and users not following proper disposal procedures. However, understanding these trends is crucial for building a sustainable digital health future.

Current Measurement Efforts

While specific data on digital health waste is limited, we can draw insights from broader e-waste statistics:

1. The Global E-Waste Monitor series, led by UNITAR and ITU, provides valuable data on overall e-waste trends.
2. Only forty-one countries currently produce their own national statistics on e-waste, with estimates made for others.

For our analysis, we will focus on two categories most relevant to digital health:

- Screens and monitors (including medical displays)
- Small IT and telecommunications equipment (including many portable medical devices)

Key Trends

1. Volume increase: Between 2010 and 2022, the volume of waste in these categories increased globally by 30 percent, from 8.1 million tons to 10.5 million tons.

2. Regional disparities

   - Developed countries saw an 11 percent increase.
   - Developing countries experienced a 48 percent increase.
   - The share of developed countries in global waste generation decreased from 48.6 to 41.5 percent.

3. Top generators (2022)

   - China (20.9 percent)
   - United States (13.9 percent)
   - European Union (12 percent)

4. Per capita generation (2022)

   - Global average: 1.33 kg
   - Developed countries: 3.25 kg
   - Developing countries: 0.93 kg
   - Least developed countries: 0.21 kg

5. Health care-specific trends

    - While exact figures for digital health waste are not available, it's estimated to be growing faster than overall e-waste due to rapid digitalization in health care.
    - Medical imaging equipment, electronic health record systems, and wearable health devices are significant contributors.

6. Data center waste

    - Rapid refresh cycles in health care data centers contribute significantly to e-waste.
    - Servers are typically replaced every three to five years for energy efficiency gains.

5.4 Sustainable Digital Health: Balancing Progress and Environmental Responsibility

The rapid digitalization of health care, while offering immense benefits, also raises concerns about overconsumption of digital health technologies. This is particularly evident in developed countries, where the frequent replacement of functional medical devices and the proliferation of digital health tools contribute significantly to e-waste generation.

Defining Sustainable Digital Health

To address this issue, we must first define what sustainable consumption looks like in the context of digital health. Drawing from Sustainable Development Goal 12, we can define sustainable digital health as

the use of digital health services and related products that respond to essential health care needs and improve quality of care while minimizing the use of natural resources, toxic materials, and the emission of waste and pollutants over the lifecycle of the technology, ensuring that future generations' health needs are not jeopardized.

In essence, sustainable digital health is about "doing more and better with less" in health care settings.

Challenges of Overconsumption in Digital Health

Several factors contribute to overconsumption in digital health:

1. Rapid technological obsolescence: The fast pace of innovation in medical technology often leads to the premature replacement of functional devices.
2. Marketing pressures: Aggressive marketing of marginally improved medical devices can drive unnecessary upgrades.
3. Data security concerns: The need to protect patient data can lead to the destruction of still-functional hardware.
4. Regulatory compliance: Changing health care regulations may require equipment upgrades even when existing technology is still functional.
5. Digital divide in health care: While developing countries struggle to acquire basic digital health infrastructure, developed countries often have multiple redundant systems.

Toward a Sustainable Digital Health Model

Moving toward sustainable digital health requires a balanced approach:

1. Moderation in high-consumption settings: Health care systems in developed countries should focus on extending the lifespan of digital health technologies and prioritizing meaningful upgrades.
2. Equitable access in underserved areas: Efforts should be made to increase access to essential digital health technologies in developing countries and underserved communities.
3. Circular economy in health care: Implementing principles of reuse, refurbishment, and recycling specifically for medical devices and health IT infrastructure.

4. Digital sufficiency in health care: Adopting a "digital sobriety" approach that prioritizes needs-based consumption of digital health technologies.
5. Lifecycle assessment: Implementing comprehensive lifecycle assessments for digital health technologies to understand and mitigate their environmental impact.

The Doughnut Model of Sustainable Digital Health

Adapting Kate Raworth's *doughnut economics* model to digital health, we can envision the following scenarios:

- Inner circle (social foundation): This represents the minimum level of digital health technology necessary to meet basic health care needs and ensure health equity.
- Outer circle (ecological ceiling): This represents the maximum level of digital health consumption that can be sustained without breaching environmental limits.
- The "sweet spot": The area between these circles represents sustainable digital health—where health care needs are met without exceeding planetary boundaries.

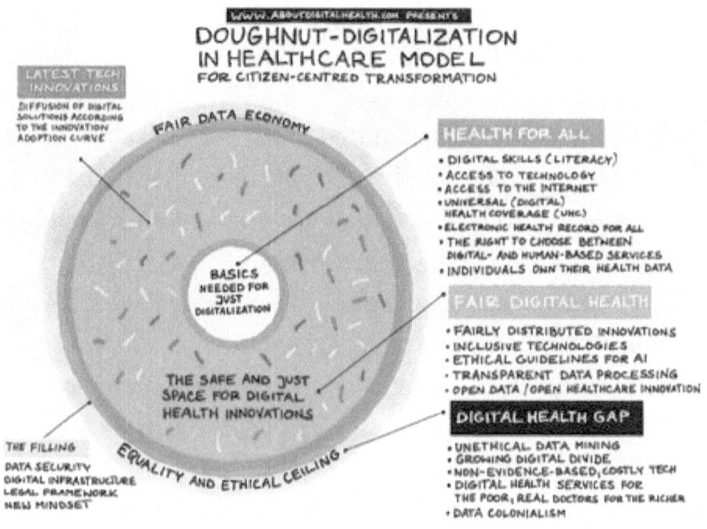

The goal of sustainable digital health is to find the balance between insufficient digitalization, which fails to meet health care needs, and overconsumption, which strains environmental resources. The following are among the ways to find such balance:

- Prioritizing essential digital health technologies in underserved areas
- Implementing sufficiency-oriented practices in well-equipped health care systems
- Developing technologies with longer lifespans and easier upgradeability
- Fostering a culture of responsible consumption in health care technology

By embracing these principles, the health care sector can lead the way in demonstrating how technological advancement can coexist with environmental stewardship, truly embodying the ethos of "First, do no harm" on both individual and planetary scales.

Challenges and Considerations

- Overconsumption: In developed countries, frequent replacement of functional medical devices driven by aggressive marketing of marginal upgrades contributes to waste.
- Planned obsolescence: Diminishing durability and repairability of medical devices exacerbates the waste problem.
- Digital divide: While developing countries are rapidly increasing their digital health infrastructure (and associated waste), developed countries still generate significantly more waste per capita.
- Data security: Destruction of hard drives containing sensitive patient data contributes to waste generation in health care settings.
- Specialized equipment: Many digital health devices (e.g., MRI machines, robotic surgical systems) have unique disposal challenges due to their size and complexity.

Future Projections

- Overall, e-waste is projected to increase from 62 million tons in 2022 to 82 million tons in 2030.
- Digital health-related waste is likely to follow a similar growth trajectory, potentially outpacing overall e-waste growth due to increasing health care digitalization.

The rapid growth of digital health-related waste presents both challenges and opportunities for the health care sector. As we advance toward more digitalized health care, it's crucial to implement strategies that balance technological progress with environmental responsibility. This includes:

1. Improving waste measurement and tracking specific to digital health technologies
2. Developing circular economy approaches for medical devices
3. Implementing responsible consumption practices in health care settings
4. Addressing the digital health divide while mitigating excessive waste generation

By understanding and addressing these trends, we can work toward a digital health future that truly embodies the principle of "First, do no harm"—not just for patients but for our planet as well.

5.5 Factors Driving the Growth of Digital Health-Related Waste

The rapid increase in digital health-related waste can be attributed to several key factors:

1. Accelerated digitalization of health care

    - increasing adoption of electronic health records, telemedicine platforms, and AI-powered diagnostic tools

- growing use of wearable health devices and remote patient-monitoring systems
- expansion of health IT infrastructure to support data-driven health care

2. Economic and regulatory pressures

   - declining prices of digital health technologies, making frequent upgrades more feasible
   - regulatory requirements driving regular updates of medical equipment
   - competitive pressures in health care pushing for the latest technologies

3. Limited awareness

   - insufficient understanding among health care providers and patients about the environmental impact of digital health waste
   - lack of knowledge about proper disposal methods for medical electronic devices

4. Linear production model

   - prevalence of a "take, make, use, dispose" approach in medical technology manufacturing
   - insufficient implementation of circular economy principles in health care technology design

5. Repair and upgrade challenges

   - the complexity of medical devices often preventing easy repairs or component replacements
   - proprietary designs limiting third-party repairs of health care equipment
   - high costs associated with repairing sophisticated medical technologies

6. Shortened life cycles

    - rapid advancements in medical technology rendering older equipment obsolete
    - "fast tech" culture in health care, with frequent upgrades of digital health tools
    - commercial practices encouraging regular replacements of medical devices

7. Data security concerns

    - need to destroy or replace devices containing sensitive patient data
    - difficulty in securely wiping data from certain types of medical equipment

8. Obsolescence in digital health

    a. Technical obsolescence
       - medical devices becoming nonfunctional due to irreplaceable components

    b. Software obsolescence
       - incompatibility issues with newer health IT systems
       - discontinued support for older software versions in medical equipment

    c. Regulatory obsolescence
       - Changes in health care regulations requiring equipment upgrades

    d. Perceived obsolescence
       - marketing pressures in promoting the latest medical technologies
       - Health care providers seeking cutting-edge equipment to attract patients

9. Intensive use in health care settings

    - continuous operation of medical equipment leading to faster wear and tear
    - high-performance requirements in critical care settings necessitating frequent upgrades

10. Lack of standardization

    - proprietary connectors and accessories limiting interoperability between different manufacturers' equipment
    - diversity of health care IT systems complicating long-term use and integration

Addressing these factors requires a multifaceted approach involving health care providers, technology manufacturers, policymakers, and patients. Strategies should focus on extending device lifespans, improving repairability, enhancing interoperability, and fostering a culture of sustainable consumption in health care technology.

By understanding and tackling these drivers of digital health waste, we can work toward a more sustainable health care future that balances technological advancement with environmental responsibility, truly embodying the principle of "First, do no harm."

5.6 Environmental, Health, and Social Impacts of Digital Health Waste

The rapid growth of digital health technologies, while offering immense benefits for patient care, also presents significant challenges in terms of waste management. Digital health-related waste contains hazardous materials that, if not properly handled, can have detrimental effects on both the environment and human health.

Hazardous Materials and Their Impacts

1. Toxic components: Digital health devices often contain heavy metals and substances such as arsenic, cadmium, lead, and mercury, as well as persistent organic pollutants.
2. Environmental contamination: Improper disposal can lead to the release of these toxins into soil, water, and air, affecting ecosystems and biodiversity.
3. Health risks: Exposure to these materials can cause a range of health issues, including neurodevelopmental disorders, renal and cardiovascular damage, reproductive issues, and various forms of cancer.

Informal Waste Management in Developing Countries

In many developing regions, a significant portion of digital health waste is handled in informal settings, presenting both opportunities and challenges:

1. Economic opportunities: Informal recycling provides livelihoods for workers and small businesses, contributing to poverty reduction and potentially narrowing digital health divides by making refurbished equipment more affordable.
2. Inefficient resource recovery: Suboptimal processes often lead to inefficient extraction of valuable materials from medical devices.
3. Occupational hazards: Workers in informal settings frequently lack proper safety equipment and knowledge about handling hazardous materials.
4. Gender disparities: Women in the informal e-waste sector often face discrimination, occupying lower-paying positions with limited growth opportunities.

Vulnerable Populations

Certain groups are particularly at risk from the impacts of digital health waste:

1. Children: They may be involved in informal waste processing due to their smaller hands, risking exposure to toxic materials during crucial developmental stages.
2. Pregnant women: Exposure can lead to adverse neonatal outcomes, including increased rates of stillbirth and premature birth.
3. Local communities: Areas near informal recycling sites may face increased air, water, and soil pollution, affecting overall community health.

Health Care–Specific Concerns

1. Data security: Improper disposal of digital health devices can lead to breaches of sensitive patient information.
2. Loss of valuable resources: Inefficient recycling processes result in the loss of rare and valuable materials used in advanced medical technologies.
3. Regulatory challenges: The complex nature of medical devices often requires specialized disposal methods, which may not be available in all regions.

Balancing Short-Term Needs and Long-Term Sustainability

In developing countries, there's a tension between

- the immediate need to provide livelihoods for those involved in informal e-waste processing and
- the long-term imperative to protect public health and the environment from the hazards of improper waste management

Moving Forward

To address these challenges while harnessing the benefits of digital health, we need the following:

1. Improved waste management policies: Developing comprehensive, health care–specific e-waste management strategies

2. Education and training: Providing proper training for those handling digital health waste, both in formal and informal sectors
3. Sustainable design: Encouraging the development of medical technologies with reduced toxic components and improved recyclability.
4. Global cooperation: Fostering international collaboration to address the transboundary nature of e-waste flows in health care.
5. Investment in infrastructure: Developing proper recycling facilities capable of handling specialized medical electronic waste.

By addressing these environmental, health, and social impacts, we can ensure that our pursuit of advanced digital health solutions truly adheres to the principle of "First, do no harm," protecting not just individual patients but also the broader communities and environments in which health care operates.

5.7 Circular Digital Health Economy: Transforming Waste into Resources

The rapid growth of digital health-related waste is becoming a global concern, affecting both developed and developing countries. While developed nations still produce significantly more waste per capita, developing countries are rapidly digitalizing their health care systems, contributing to an increasing share of this waste. However, the persistent digital divide in health care also reflects an uneven capacity to manage the associated waste.

When digital health waste is properly managed in a safe and environmentally sound manner, the risks to both human health and the environment can be minimized or avoided. Therefore, it's crucial to strengthen formal systems for collecting and processing digital health waste. This approach not only mitigates risks, it also promotes more efficient recovery of valuable resources embedded in medical technologies.

Management of Digital Health-Related Waste: Beyond Recycling and Resource Recovery

The rapid increase in digital health-related waste presents significant challenges for its management, particularly in developing economies. While there has been progress in formal collection and recycling of electronic waste, including medical devices and health IT equipment, these efforts have not kept pace with the growing volume of waste generated.

Global Trends in Digital Health Waste Management

- Collection rates: Globally, less than a quarter of digital health-related waste is formally collected, leaving over three-quarters undocumented and potentially mismanaged.
- Regional disparities: Developed economies have significantly higher collection rates (averaging 46.8 percent) compared to developing economies (averaging 7.5 percent).
- Legislative framework: While eighty-two countries have e-waste policies or legislation in place, only 25 percent of developing countries are covered, highlighting a significant policy gap.

Challenges in Managing Digital Health Waste

- Complexity of medical devices: Advanced health care technologies often contain complex alloys and materials, complicating recycling processes.
- Limited recycling technology: The availability of technology capable of recycling sophisticated medical equipment remains limited.
- Economic viability: The high cost of recycling certain components in medical devices can outweigh the benefits.
- Insufficient Infrastructure: Many regions lack proper collection and treatment facilities for digital health waste.
- Worker training: There's a shortage of trained personnel capable of handling digital health waste safely, particularly in informal sectors.

- Lack of formal collection systems: Many regions lack the infrastructure to handle digital health waste sustainably.
- Data security: The need to protect patient data complicates the disposal and recycling of medical electronic devices.
- Consumer awareness: Health care providers and patients often lack awareness of proper disposal methods for digital health devices.

Beyond Recycling: A Holistic Approach

While recycling and resource recovery are important, they should not be the sole focus of digital health waste management. A more comprehensive approach is needed.

- Waste reduction: Prioritize strategies to reduce the overall volume of digital health waste generated.
- Extended producer responsibility (EPR): Implement policies that make health care technology manufacturers responsible for the entire lifecycle of their products.
- Design for sustainability: Encourage the development of medical devices that are easier to repair, upgrade, and recycle.
- Circular economy principles: Adopt a circular approach in health care technology, emphasizing reuse, refurbishment, and remanufacturing before recycling.
- Health and environmental standards: Ensure that e-waste legislation in health care addresses both environmental protection and occupational safety.
- Value capture in developing countries: Develop policies that enable developing nations to capture more value from digital health waste management activities.

To address the growing challenge of digital health waste, a multifaceted approach is essential. This includes accelerating the adoption of comprehensive waste policies, particularly in developing countries, while simultaneously increasing investment in proper collection and treatment infrastructure.

Equally important is the need to invest in research and innovation to develop new technologies capable of recycling complex medical devices. Given the global nature of this issue, fostering international collaboration is crucial to effectively manage transboundary waste flows.

Finally, implementing education and awareness programs for health care providers and patients about proper disposal methods is vital. By integrating these strategies—policy development, infrastructure investment, technological innovation, global cooperation, and education—we can create a more sustainable approach to digital health waste management, ensuring that our efforts to improve health care don't come at the cost of environmental degradation.

While recycling and resource recovery are important components of digital health waste management, they are not sufficient on their own. A more holistic approach that prioritizes waste reduction, sustainable design, and circular economy principles is essential. By addressing the entire life cycle of digital health technologies, from design to disposal, we can create a more sustainable health care system that truly embodies the principle of "First, do no harm"—not just for patients but for our planet as well.

Circular Economy in Digital Health: Beyond Recycling

The circular economy approach for digital health technologies offers a comprehensive alternative to the traditional linear model of production and consumption. This approach considers the entire lifecycle of medical devices and health IT equipment, from design and manufacturing to use and end-of-life management.

Key Elements of Circular Economy in Digital Health

Sustainable design. Developing medical devices and health IT equipment with longevity, repairability, and recyclability in mind

Reducing. Health care providers must rethink how they can meet patient needs with minimal environmental impact. This may involve the following solutions:

- using functioning medical equipment for longer periods
- adopting "medical equipment as a service" models
- refurbishment and remanufacturing: giving new life to used medical equipment through professional refurbishment processes.
- secondary markets: promoting the resale and redistribution of refurbished medical devices to health care facilities with limited resources
- implementing AI-driven resource optimization to reduce unnecessary device usage

Refusing. This sustainable choice involves:

- declining unnecessary upgrades or replacements of medical devices
- avoiding products with hazardous substances
- opting out of bundled purchases that include unnecessary equipment

Direct reuse. In health care, this could mean:

- redeploying medical devices to different departments or facilities
- donating functional equipment to underserved health care facilities
- establishing equipment sharing programs between health care providers

Repairing. This is crucial in health care but faces unique challenges:

- Many medical devices are not designed for easy repair.
- Access to repair manuals and components is often restricted.
- Specialized repairers may be costly or scarce.

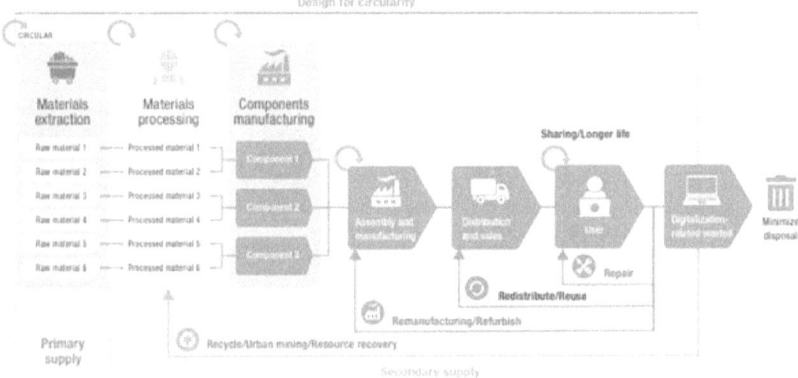

Circular Economy for Digital Solutions

Benefits of Circular Approaches in Health Care

- Environmental: Reduces the demand for raw materials and minimizes e-waste generation
- Economic: Creates new business opportunities in device refurbishment and recycling
- Social: Improves access to medical technologies in underserved areas through refurbished equipment

Market Trends

The market for circular economy activities in health care is growing rapidly:

- The global market for medical device recycling is projected to reach $9.5 billion by 2027.
- Refurbished medical equipment market is expected to grow at a CAGR of 10.5 percent from 2021 to 2028.
- Demand for repaired and refurbished medical devices is increasing, particularly in developing countries.

Challenges and Opportunities

- Data security: Ensuring proper data erasure from medical devices before refurbishment or recycling.
- Regulatory compliance: Navigating complex regulations around the reuse of medical equipment.
- Technological obsolescence: Balancing the need for cutting-edge technology with sustainable practices.
- Supply chain complexity: Developing reverse logistics systems for collecting and processing used medical devices.

To fully harness the potential of the circular economy in digital health, a multifaceted approach is essential. This includes implementing supportive regulations for the repair, refurbishment, and recycling of medical devices; fostering collaborative partnerships among health care providers, manufacturers, and recycling firms; investing in innovative technologies that simplify the disassembly and recycling of complex medical equipment; and educating health care professionals about the benefits and practices of circular economy principles in their field. By integrating these strategic actions, the health care sector can create a more sustainable ecosystem that maximizes the lifespan and value of digital health technologies while minimizing waste and environmental impact.

The circular economy approach in digital health offers a pathway to more sustainable health care delivery. By extending the life of medical devices, promoting refurbishment, and improving recycling practices, the health care sector can significantly reduce its environmental footprint while maintaining high standards of patient care. This shift not only addresses the growing e-waste challenge, it also aligns with the broader goal of creating a more sustainable and equitable health care system.

5.8 Conclusion

The rapid global digitalization of health care is leading to an increasing demand for digital health equipment and the minerals used to manufacture it. This surge in demand puts significant pressure on the world's primary supply of minerals and metals, a challenge exacerbated by the broader transition to low-carbon technologies.

While recycling digital health-related waste and recovering materials through urban mining can help alleviate some of this pressure, these efforts alone are insufficient to address the environmental impacts of producing and disposing of medical electronic equipment. A more comprehensive approach is needed, embracing the full spectrum of circular economy principles in health care.

The circular digital health economy offers a pathway to both environmental and economic benefits. It can contribute to the sound management of health care e-waste, reduce the demand for natural resources, and create new economic opportunities, including in developing countries. However, realizing these benefits requires a fundamental shift in mindset regarding the consumption and production of health care technologies.

Key considerations for moving toward a more circular approach in digital health include:

1. Stakeholder collaboration: Joint action and responsibility from all stakeholders in the health care ecosystem is crucial. This includes medical device manufacturers, health care providers, policymakers, and patients.
2. Sustainable design: Manufacturers must prioritize designing digital health equipment for circularity, ensuring devices last longer and can be easily repaired, disassembled, and recycled.
3. Consumer behavior: Health care providers and patients need to reconsider their approach to digital health technologies, favoring

longer device lifespans and making conscious decisions to use more sustainable equipment.
4. Policy support: Appropriate policies at the national, regional, and international levels are needed to create enabling factors for circular economy practices in health care. These policies should be based on the principle of common but differentiated responsibilities, considering the varying capabilities and needs of different countries.
5. Improved measurement: Strengthening the measurement of digital health-related waste and its international flows is crucial. Better data is essential for informed policymaking and understanding the dynamics of international trade in health care e-waste.
6. Digital tools for circularity: Leveraging digital technologies, such as digital product passports for medical devices, can enhance the tracking of materials and products, enabling more informed consumption decisions and effective policies.
7. Balancing innovation and sustainability: The health care sector must find ways to continue advancing medical technologies while minimizing environmental impact.

Moving toward a circular digital health economy is not just an environmental imperative but a crucial step in ensuring that our efforts to improve health care through digitalization truly adhere to the principle of "First, do no harm." By embracing these circular economy principles, the health care sector can lead the way in demonstrating how technological advancement can coexist with environmental stewardship, creating a more sustainable and equitable health care future for all.

Chapter 6

Digital Health Platforms and Environmental Sustainability

6.1 Introduction

While the preceding chapters focused on the three phases of the life cycle of digital health technologies, this chapter discusses a specific application of these technologies: digital health platforms. We turn our attention to the indirect implications of health care digitalization on the environment, which can be both positive and negative.

As stressed earlier, assessing these indirect effects is even more challenging than measuring the direct environmental footprint of digital health technologies. However, understanding these impacts is crucial as we strive to build a health care system that truly embodies the principle of "First, do no harm"—not just for individual patients but for our planet as well.

This chapter has a particular focus on patient-facing digital health platforms, including the following:

- Telemedicine platforms
- Remote patient monitoring systems

- Digital health marketplaces
- Personal health record management systems
- AI-powered health diagnostic tools

We will explore how these platforms can be designed and operated in the most environmentally sustainable manner possible.

Digitalization has profoundly impacted health care delivery and access. Accelerated by the COVID-19 pandemic, more patients and health care providers are turning to digital platforms for health services, consultations, and medical information.

"Digital health platforms" refer to all systems where health services or information are ordered, delivered, or managed over a computer network (e.g., the internet). These platforms can involve various stakeholders, including health care providers, patients, insurers, and health technology companies. Digital health transactions often cross international borders, with providers and patients potentially located in different countries.

The shift to digital health platforms brings both opportunities and challenges. It can transform health care processes, improve access to specialized care, and open up new opportunities for health care innovation. Patients can benefit from greater choice, convenience, and potentially lower costs. However, challenges related to digital infrastructure, data security, regulatory frameworks, and digital literacy pose critical barriers to engaging in and benefiting from digital health, especially in low-income countries.

Digital health platforms have potential implications for environmental sustainability that are both positive and negative. For example, telemedicine consultations can be more energy-efficient than traveling to a physical clinic, potentially reducing GHG emissions. Some medical services can now be delivered digitally, enabling dematerialization of certain aspects of health care. On the other hand, increased access to health care through digital platforms may lead to higher overall resource consumption, increased energy use for data centers, and potential e-waste from medical devices.

The primary emphasis of this chapter is on the indirect environmental effects of health care digitalization through digital health platforms. We will explore the environmental impact linked to the following:

- Changes in patient travel patterns
- Energy usage across the digital health infrastructure
- Potential increases in medical device production and disposal
- Changes in health care delivery models and their resource implications

While this chapter focuses primarily on patient-facing digital health platforms (analogous to B2C e-commerce), we will also touch upon provider-to-provider telemedicine (similar to B2B) and peer-to-peer health communities (akin to C2C).

The chapter is structured as follows:

Section 1 presents recent trends in digital health platform adoption.

Section 2 provides a comparative review of the environmental impact of digital health platforms versus traditional in-person health care delivery.

Section 3 explores measures to reduce negative environmental impacts and build more sustainable digital health ecosystems.

Section 4 discusses the potential for digital health platforms to enable circular economy principles in health care.

The final section provides specific recommendations to stakeholders on how to make digital health platforms more environmentally sustainable.

By examining these aspects, we aim to provide a comprehensive understanding of how digital health platforms can be leveraged to improve patient care while minimizing environmental impact, truly embodying the principle of "First, do no harm."

6.2 Digital Health Platform Trends, Opportunities, and Risks

The proliferation of the internet has rapidly and fundamentally transformed health care delivery. From virtually nonexistent in the early 1990s, digital health platforms have surged in popularity, with an estimated 2.5 billion people using digital health services globally by 2023.

Since 2010, the adoption of digital health platforms has greatly increased in many countries, further accelerated by the COVID-19 pandemic. However, the extent of engagement varies considerably. In countries with the highest uptake, more than 80 percent of the population uses digital health services; in most of the least developed countries (LDCs), that share remains below 10 percent.

The global digital health market is estimated to reach $550 billion by 2027, up from $175 billion in 2019. For example, in the United States, the telemedicine market grew from $38 billion in 2019 to an estimated $112 billion in 2023.

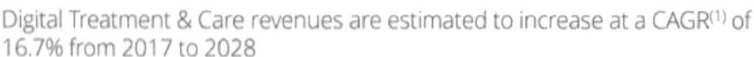

Digital Treatment & Care revenues are estimated to increase at a CAGR[(1)] of 16.7% from 2017 to 2028

Market Size: Global

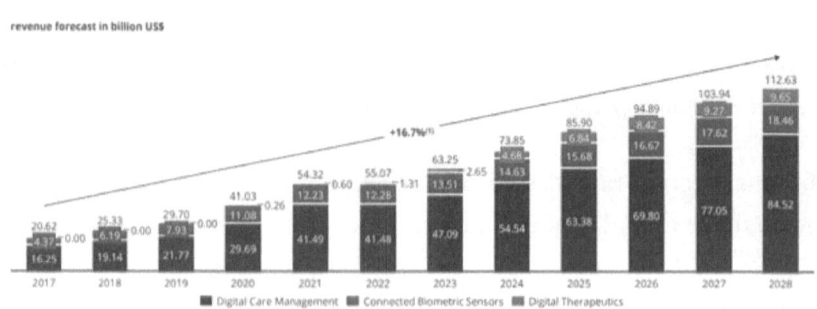

Digital health platform usage in developed economies far exceeds that in developing economies. While the latter account for around 40 percent of the global population, their share of digital health market value is at most 25 percent, suggesting significant growth potential.

Patients can engage with digital health platforms through various channels, including:

- Dedicated telemedicine platforms
- Hospital or clinic-specific patient portals
- Third-party health marketplaces
- Mobile health apps
- AI-powered health chatbots

Many health care providers now offer "omnichannel" care, combining in-person visits with digital consultations to meet patient needs.

Large technology companies have emerged as key players in the digital health landscape, often partnering with traditional health care providers. This market concentration raises questions about data privacy and equitable access to health care, as well as presents opportunities for these companies to lead in making digital health environmentally sustainable.

Digital health platforms can offer opportunities for the following scenarios:

- improved access to health care in underserved areas
- more flexible and efficient health care delivery
- empowerment of patients through better health information and self-management tools
- new opportunities for health care professionals, including remote work options

However, these opportunities must be viewed against a backdrop of highly uneven levels of digital health readiness. Future trajectories and the ability of developing countries and LDCs to unlock the potential of digital health for all depends on policy actions that address the following situations:

- digital infrastructure and connectivity
- health IT workforce development
- regulatory frameworks for digital health
- data privacy and security concerns
- interoperability of health information systems

In addition to these challenges, the environmental impact of expanding digital health platforms must be considered. This impact varies depending on factors such as the following:

- energy consumption of data centers hosting health information
- changes in patient travel patterns for health care
- production and disposal of digital health devices
- potential for more efficient resource use in health care delivery through AI and data analytics

Each component of the digital health ecosystem carries potential environmental risks that can have adverse impacts on biodiversity, energy consumption, and resource use. While research on these impacts is mainly available from developed countries, understanding the environmental footprint of digital health is of growing relevance for countries at all levels of development.

As we move forward, it's crucial that the expansion of digital health platforms aligns with environmental sustainability goals, truly embodying the principle of "First, do no harm" for both patient health and planetary well-being.

6.3 Environmental Effects of Digital Health Platforms vs. Traditional Health Care Delivery: A Comparative Analysis

How has the shift from traditional health care delivery to digital health platforms impacted the environment? This section reviews findings from studies that have empirically assessed the environmental sustainability of digital and traditional health care options, focusing on GHG emissions, energy use, and resource consumption patterns. Most data comes from developed countries, with limited studies from developing nations.

6.3.1. Factors Impacting Environmental Sustainability in Health Care

Different parameters related to infrastructure, transportation, equipment, and patient behavior affect the environmental footprint of both digital and traditional health care delivery.

A. Infrastructure and Energy Use

Digital health platforms rely heavily on data centers and IT infrastructure, which consume significant energy. However, they may reduce the need for large physical health care facilities. Traditional health care delivery requires energy-intensive hospital buildings and medical equipment.

A study in the US found that telemedicine could reduce carbon emissions by up to 70 percent compared to in-person visits, primarily due to reduced patient travel and lower energy use in physical facilities. However, the energy consumption of data centers supporting telemedicine services needs consideration.

B. Medical Equipment and Waste Generation

Digital health may reduce the need for certain disposable medical supplies used in face-to-face consultations. However, it can increase electronic waste from devices and sensors used in remote patient monitoring.

A UK study found that remote monitoring of chronic conditions could reduce medical waste by 30 percent compared to traditional care models. However, the lifecycle environmental impact of wearable devices and sensors needs further research.

C. Transportation and patient travel

Digital health platforms significantly reduce patient travel, potentially lowering transport-related emissions. A study in Canada estimated that widespread adoption of telemedicine could reduce health care–related travel emissions by up to 40 percent. However, the environmental benefits can vary based on local transportation infrastructure and the energy sources powering digital devices and networks.

D. Patient behavior and resource consumption

Digital health platforms may influence patient behavior in ways that affect resource consumption. For instance, easier access to health care through telemedicine might increase overall health care utilization, potentially leading to more prescriptions and medical interventions.

A study in Sweden found that while telemedicine reduced travel-related emissions, it led to a 15 percent increase in prescription rates, highlighting the complex relationship between accessibility and resource use in health care.

As with other assessments of secondary environmental effects of digitalization, it's challenging to draw definitive conclusions on whether traditional or digital health care delivery is preferable from an environmental sustainability perspective. The environmental footprint depends on many factors, and comparing results from various studies is difficult due to the absence of a common assessment approach.

Ultimately, the issue is not so much whether digital health is more or less environmentally friendly than traditional health care delivery. In many countries, patients and providers use both channels. However, given the observed environmental risks and benefits of digital health, it's essential to consider how to ensure that digital health platforms are as environmentally sustainable as possible.

Given the particularly scarce evidence on the environmental impact of digital health in developing countries, it's important to build a stronger knowledge base for these regions. Future research should focus on the following areas:

1. Comprehensive lifecycle assessments of digital health technologies
2. Energy efficiency of health IT infrastructure in different geographical contexts
3. The impact of digital health on overall health care resource consumption patterns
4. Strategies for minimizing e-waste from digital health devices

By understanding these factors, we can work toward a digital health future that not only improves patient care but also minimizes environmental impact, truly embodying the principle of "First, do no harm."

6.4 Making Digital Health More Environmentally Sustainable

The environmental impacts of digital health can be influenced through various approaches. Government policy and legislation play a crucial role, as does the adoption of more inclusive and environmentally sustainable digital health practices and business models. Encouraging health care providers and patients to be better informed and to change their behavior is also essential. Large digital health platforms have a significant responsibility to foster more environmentally sustainable practices.

The design of policy measures and transformative actions across the digital health ecosystem—from technology development and infrastructure to service delivery and patient engagement—can be improved. The following are the aims of these efforts:

1. Optimize resource use in health care delivery
2. Cut GHG emissions associated with digital health infrastructure
3. Reduce unnecessary digital interactions and data generation
4. Lower e-waste from medical devices and health IT equipment
5. Drive sustainable development in the health care sector

Making digital health more environmentally sustainable can create interconnected benefits across several Sustainable Development Goals, including the following:

- Goal 3 (good health and well-being)
- Goal 7 (affordable and clean energy)
- Goal 9 (industry, innovation, and infrastructure)
- Goal 11 (sustainable cities and communities)
- Goal 12 (responsible consumption and production)
- Goal 13 (climate action)

This section focuses on how to mitigate risks and harness opportunities for improving environmental sustainability in digital health. Attention is given to the following:

1. Government policies and regulations
2. Actions by digital health platforms and health care providers
3. Initiatives by health technology companies
4. Engagement of patients and health care consumers
5. Role of medical professionals in promoting sustainable digital health practices

By addressing these areas, we can work toward a digital health future that not only improves patient care but also minimizes environmental impact. This holistic approach ensures that as we advance health care through technology, we truly embody the principle of "First, do no harm"—extending it from individual patient care to the health of our planet.

The following subsections will explore specific strategies and best practices for each of these areas, providing a roadmap for building a more sustainable digital health ecosystem.

6.4.1 Reducing the Environmental Impact of Digital Health Infrastructure

A. Optimizing Data Centers and Health IT Infrastructure

There are multiple ways to reduce the environmental footprint of health care data centers and IT infrastructure:

- Renewable energy: Implement renewable energy sources, such as solar panels, to power health care data centers. For example, Kaiser Permanente has installed solar panels at many of its facilities, significantly reducing its carbon footprint.
- Energy-efficient technologies: Utilize energy-efficient servers, storage systems, and cooling technologies. Epic Systems, a major electronic health record provider, has implemented advanced cooling systems in its data centers, reducing energy consumption by up to 40 percent.
- Smart resource management: Implement AI-driven resource allocation systems to optimize server usage and reduce idle energy consumption. IBM's Watson for Health uses such systems to manage its cloud-based health care services more efficiently.

B. Minimizing E-Waste from Medical Devices

Digital health generates significant electronic waste. Minimizing this impact includes the following strategies:

- Sustainable device design: Encourage manufacturers to design medical devices and wearables for longevity, repairability, and recyclability. For instance, Philips has committed to making all its medical equipment recyclable or reusable by 2025.
- Recycling programs: Establish comprehensive recycling programs for medical electronic devices. Medtronic, a leading medical device company, has implemented a take-back program for its devices, ensuring proper recycling and disposal.
- Refurbishment initiatives: Promote the refurbishment and reuse of medical equipment. Organizations like MedShare refurbish and distribute used medical equipment to underserved health care facilities, extending device lifecycles.

C. Sustainable Telemedicine Practices

As telemedicine grows, so does its potential environmental impact. Minimizing its impact includes these strategies:

- Energy-efficient video conferencing: Utilize low-bandwidth, energy-efficient video-conferencing technologies. Zoom Healthcare, for example, has implemented features to reduce bandwidth usage in telemedicine consultations.
- Optimized scheduling: Implement AI-driven scheduling systems to reduce unnecessary virtual appointments and optimize provider time. Babylon Health uses such systems to streamline its telemedicine services.
- Patient education: Educate patients on the environmental benefits of telemedicine compared to in-person visits, encouraging its use when appropriate.

First, Do No Harm | 113

D. Green Health Information Exchange (HIE)

Efficient health information exchange can reduce redundant tests and procedures, indirectly reducing environmental impact:

- Interoperability standards: Promote widespread adoption of interoperability standards to reduce data duplication and associated energy consumption. The Fast Healthcare Interoperability Resources (FHIR) standard is a step in this direction.
- Cloud-based solutions: Encourage the use of cloud-based HIE solutions, which can be more energy-efficient than on-premise systems. Companies like Google Cloud Healthcare API offer such solutions.

By adopting these sustainable practices and optimizing digital health infrastructure, the health care sector can significantly reduce its carbon footprint and environmental impact. From a broader sustainable development perspective, these efforts should be accompanied by measures to ensure data privacy, security, and equitable access to digital health services.

Implementing these strategies requires collaboration between health care providers, technology companies, policymakers, and patients. By working together, we can create a digital health ecosystem that improves patient care while minimizing harm to our planet, truly embodying the principle of "First, do no harm."

E. Toward More Sustainable Digital Health Delivery

The rapid growth of digital health services is placing increased pressure on data centers and network infrastructure, contributing significantly to the health care sector's carbon footprint. The digital health sector, including telemedicine and remote patient monitoring, accounts for an estimated 4 to 5 percent of global health care-related emissions. As demand for these services grows, there's an urgent need to address their environmental impact.

Fast and frequent digital interactions, driven by patient demand and competition among providers, often result in inefficient use of computing resources and increased energy consumption. For instance, providers offering instant telemedicine consultations may maintain underutilized servers, leading to unnecessary energy use and emissions.

Without effective intervention, emissions from digital health services are projected to increase by 40 percent by 2030. However, with ecosystem-wide changes, we could reduce emissions by 30 percent and cut operational costs by 25 percent compared to a "business as usual" scenario.

For example:

- Cloud migration: Moving health care data and services to energy-efficient cloud providers could reduce emissions by up to 20 percent.
- AI-optimized resource allocation: Implementing AI systems to manage computing resources more efficiently could cut energy use by 15 to 25 percent.
- Edge computing: Deploying edge computing for certain health care applications could reduce data center energy consumption by 10 to 5 percent.

Sustainable Digital Health Strategies

1. Green data centers: Health care providers should prioritize partnering with data centers powered by renewable energy. For example, Kaiser Permanente has committed to carbon-neutral operations, including its digital health services.
2. Efficient telemedicine platforms: Develop and use video-conferencing solutions optimized for low energy consumption. Zoom Health, for instance, has introduced energy-saving features for telemedicine consultations.

3. Smart scheduling: Implement AI-driven scheduling systems to optimize virtual appointment slots and reduce idle server time. Companies like Babylon Health are pioneering such approaches.
4. Local data processing: Where possible, process and store health data locally to reduce long-distance data transmission and associated energy costs.
5. Energy-efficient devices: Promote the use of energy-efficient devices for remote patient monitoring. For example, Withings has developed low-power wearables for continuous health tracking.

Policy Innovations

1. Green digital health certifications: Introduce certifications for environmentally sustainable digital health services.
2. Emissions reporting: Mandate regular reporting of carbon emissions from digital health operations.
3. Research funding: Allocate funds for developing energy-efficient health care AI and telemedicine technologies.

Global Initiatives

Several organizations are leading the way in sustainable digital health:

- The NHS in the UK has committed to net-zero emissions, including its digital services, by 2040.
- Teladoc Health has partnered with renewable energy providers to power its telemedicine platform.
- In India, Practo is using solar-powered clinics for its hybrid telemedicine services in rural areas.

The transition to sustainable digital health delivery offers a promising pathway for reducing health care's environmental impact. However, its effectiveness depends on widespread adoption of renewable energy and the development of more efficient technologies. As we advance digital health solutions, we must ensure that our efforts to improve patient care don't come at the cost of environmental harm, truly embodying the principle of "First, do no harm."

E. Optimizing Digital Health Interactions and Reducing Unnecessary Usage

As digital health services become more prevalent, there is a growing need to optimize interactions and reduce unnecessary usage to minimize environmental impact. In 2022, it was estimated that unnecessary digital health interactions resulted in over $300 billion in wasted health care spending globally, with associated environmental costs.

Understanding the factors driving excessive digital health usage is crucial for developing targeted solutions. These are among the key drivers:

1. Patient anxiety leading to frequent check-ins
2. Poorly designed user interfaces that cause confusion
3. Lack of clarity in telemedicine consultations necessitating follow-ups
4. Overuse of remote monitoring devices generating excessive data

To address these issues, health care providers and digital health companies could consider the following solutions:

1. Implementing AI-driven triage systems to prioritize digital health interactions
2. Improving user-interface design to reduce confusion and unnecessary logins
3. Enhancing telemedicine consultation protocols to minimize follow-ups
4. Optimizing remote monitoring thresholds to reduce data overload

Some digital health providers are already taking steps in this direction:

- Teladoc Health has introduced a "smart scheduling" system that determines whether a follow-up video consultation is necessary or if asynchronous messaging would suffice.

- Babylon Health uses AI chatbots for initial patient triage, reducing unnecessary live consultations.
- Livongo has implemented adaptive monitoring thresholds for chronic conditions, minimizing alert fatigue for both patients and providers.

Legislative and Regulatory Measures

While digital health regulations aim to protect patient rights and improve care quality, they should also consider environmental sustainability. For example:

- The EU's proposed Ecodesign for Sustainable Digital Health Products Regulation aims to make digital health devices more durable, repairable, and energy efficient.
- Some countries are introducing carbon footprint disclosure requirements for digital health services.

Practical Steps for Digital Health Providers

1. End "always-on" services: Implement smart power management for devices and services when not in active use.
2. Optimize data storage: Use efficient data compression and storage techniques to reduce server energy consumption.
3. Promote asynchronous communication: Encourage the use of secure messaging over video calls when appropriate.
4. Invest in sustainable technology: Prioritize energy-efficient servers and renewable energy for data centers.

By adopting these practices, digital health providers can reduce unnecessary system usage, lowering energy consumption and improving overall efficiency. However, it's crucial to balance these measures with ensuring patient access to care when needed.

Optimizing digital health interactions is not just about reducing costs; it's about minimizing the environmental footprint of health care technology. As we advance digital health solutions, we must ensure that our efforts to improve patient care don't come at an unnecessary cost to the environment. This approach truly embodies the principle of "First, do no harm"—extending it from individual patient care to the health of our planet.

F. Influencing Patient and Provider Behavior in Digital Health

Different patient needs and health care provider behaviors can have unintended negative environmental effects on digital health. For instance, the convenience of telemedicine and remote monitoring can lead to the overuse of these services, contributing to increased energy consumption and electronic waste.

Concerns have grown about the development of a "hyperconnected health culture" where patients and providers rely excessively on digital health tools, even when not clinically necessary. This trend can contribute to increased energy consumption, data-center loads, and unnecessary production of digital health devices.

To mitigate these trends, it's crucial to encourage more responsible use of digital health services. This would include the following strategies:

1. Ethical nudging: Implement digital nudges that encourage the appropriate use of telemedicine and remote monitoring services. For example, a reminder about the environmental impact of a video consultation versus a phone call.
2. Gamification: Develop apps that reward patients for sustainable health behaviors, such as maintaining a healthy lifestyle to reduce unnecessary digital health interactions.
3. Carbon footprint calculators: Provide tools for health care providers to understand the environmental impact of their digital health practices.

4. Positive feedback loops: Offer patients insights into how their responsible use of digital health services contributes to environmental sustainability.
5. Green activations: Implement features in digital health platforms that activate more sustainable options by default, such as lower-resolution video for noncritical consultations.

When used effectively, these strategies can help patients and providers make more environmentally conscious decisions in their use of digital health services. However, it's crucial that digital health platforms employ these tools responsibly and ethically, avoiding "dark nudges" that might compromise patient care or privacy.

For example, a telemedicine platform could provide information on the carbon footprint of different consultation options (video, audio, text) at the time of booking, allowing patients to make informed decisions. Similarly, a remote patient monitoring system could use gamification to encourage patients to maintain stable health metrics, reducing the need for data-intensive continuous monitoring.

To foster more environmentally conscious behavior and protect against greenwashing, stakeholders in digital health need reliable information on the environmental sustainability of different technologies and practices. Better access to life-cycle assessment (LCA) data for digital health products and services is crucial. This information can empower health care providers and administrators to compare technologies based not just on clinical efficacy and cost but also on their environmental footprint.

Striking the right balance between leveraging digital health for improved patient outcomes and preventing overuse is key to promoting responsible use of these technologies. As we advance digital health solutions, we must ensure that our efforts to improve health care don't come at an unnecessary cost to the environment.

By adopting these strategies, the digital health sector can work toward a more sustainable future, truly embodying the principle of "First, do no harm"—extending it from individual patient care to the health of our planet.

G. Legal and Regulatory Measures in Digital Health

Alongside technological solutions and user-engagement strategies, legislation, regulations, and guidelines addressing environmental claims and sustainability in digital health are becoming increasingly important. The rapid growth of "green" marketing in digital health presents challenges for patients, health care providers, and regulatory authorities.

While the United Nations guidelines for consumer protection don't explicitly mention environmental claims in digital health, they recommend that member states "review existing consumer protection policies to accommodate the special features of electronic commerce and ensure that consumers and businesses are informed and aware of their rights and obligations in the digital marketplace." This principle can be extended to digital health services.

A survey of regulatory measures related to environmental claims in digital health revealed that most countries lack specific legislation in this area. However, many are developing educational materials to raise awareness among health care providers, patients, and digital health companies.

Some countries have taken steps to address environmental claims in digital health:

1. In the United States, the FDA has proposed guidelines for "sustainable medical devices," which include provisions for environmental claims made by digital health companies.
2. The European Union is developing a Green Digital Health directive, which would require digital health companies to substantiate environmental claims and have them verified by third parties.

3. In Australia, the Therapeutic Goods Administration has included environmental sustainability criteria in its regulatory framework for digital health technologies.

International organizations are also supporting efforts to improve the credibility of environmental claims in digital health:

1. The World Health Organization has published "Guidelines for Sustainable Digital Health," which include recommendations for communicating sustainability information to patients and health care providers.
2. The International Medical Device Regulators Forum is developing a framework for assessing the environmental impact of digital health technologies.

Green certifications for digital health are emerging as well. For instance:

1. The Green Health IT certification evaluates the energy efficiency and sustainability of health information systems.
2. The Sustainable Telemedicine label assesses the environmental impact of remote health care delivery platforms.

These initiatives aim to create a standardized approach to evaluating and communicating the environmental impact of digital health technologies. They typically consider factors such as follows:

- Energy efficiency of devices and data centers
- Use of renewable energy in operations
- E-waste management practices
- Data minimization and efficient storage
- Promotion of sustainable health care practices

As the digital health sector continues to grow, it's crucial that these regulatory measures evolve to ensure that environmental claims are truthful, substantiated, and meaningful. This will help health care providers and patients make informed decisions that consider both health outcomes and environmental impact.

By implementing these measures, the digital health industry can move toward more sustainable practices, truly embodying the principle of "First, do no harm"—not just for individual patients but for the planet as a whole.

6.5 Opportunities for Contributing to the Circular Economy and Fostering a Sharing Economy in Digital Health

Digital health platforms can play a crucial role in promoting resource efficiency and waste reduction in health care by enabling the reuse, refurbishment, and sharing of medical devices and equipment. This can facilitate the transition to circular and sharing economies in health care, helping to reduce pressure on scarce resources and increase the efficiency of health care delivery.

The following are examples of circular economy practices in digital health:

1. Medical equipment marketplaces: Platforms, like Medinas Health, that enable hospitals to buy and sell pre-owned medical equipment, extending the lifespan of devices and reducing e-waste
2. Telemedicine resource sharing: Platforms that allow health care providers to share specialist resources across multiple facilities, optimizing the use of medical expertise and reducing the need for redundant equipment
3. AI-driven predictive maintenance: Systems that use AI to predict when medical devices need maintenance, extending their lifespan and reducing unnecessary replacements
4. Digital health device refurbishment: Programs that collect, refurbish, and redistribute digital health devices like tablets and wearables, ensuring they have multiple use cycles

5. Virtual health libraries: Platforms that allow health care providers to share digital resources, like medical imaging datasets, reducing the need for redundant data storage.

These initiatives can help lessen the demand for new products and the resources required to produce them. By facilitating the trade and sharing of medical equipment and digital health resources, these platforms may extend the lifespan of products and encourage a shift toward more responsible consumption and production in health care.

For example, the Medical Devices Reuse and Recycling Initiative in the UK reported a reduction of 5,000 tons of CO_2 emissions in one year by facilitating medical equipment refurbishment and reuse, reducing the need to produce new devices.

Another way of improving sustainability is through business models that prioritize environmental and social responsibility in digital health. For instance, Healthy.io, a digital health company, not only provides home-based urinalysis tests but also implements a take-back program for its testing kits, ensuring proper recycling and reducing medical waste.

However, it's important to note that sharing systems in health care may also lead to "rebound" effects. For example, while telemedicine platforms reduce travel-related emissions, they might inadvertently increase overall health care consumption and associated energy use. Mitigating these risks requires a collective effort from all stakeholders:

1. Governments could provide incentives to digital health companies that promote circular economy practices.
2. Health care providers could partner with organizations on initiatives that reduce medical e-waste.
3. Patients can be encouraged to use digital health services responsibly and support policies that promote circularity in health care.

By leveraging these opportunities, the digital health sector can contribute significantly to the circular economy, reducing its environmental footprint while improving health care access and quality. This approach aligns with the book's core principle of "First, do no harm," extending it from patient care to environmental stewardship in health care.

6.6 An Agenda for Action in Sustainable Digital Health

This book has explored the various environmental impacts of digital health, as well as actions and measures for more sustainable practices. As digital health continues to expand, understanding its sustainability challenges is crucial. Digital health has reshaped health care delivery patterns and infrastructure, with multiple environmental effects. While precise impact assessments are hindered by data limitations, digital health presents both opportunities and risks—from data-center operations to device manufacturing, telemedicine services, and patient behavior.

Making digital health more environmentally sustainable requires collaborative efforts from governments, health care providers, technology companies, and patients. Initiatives should focus on responsible and sustainable sourcing of medical devices, energy-efficient data centers, adopting renewable energy, eco-friendly device design, and sustainable health care consumption patterns.

Drawn from the discussion in this book, including examples of good practice, are the following recommendations for different stakeholders:

1. Promoting better digital health practices

    Governments and health care providers have complementary roles in advancing environmental sustainability in digital health:

    What governments can do:

    - Establish regulatory frameworks for sustainable digital health technologies

- Provide incentives for health care providers to adopt eco-friendly digital solutions
- Engage in international cooperation to set global standards for sustainable digital health

What health care providers and technology companies can do:

- Drive innovation in energy-efficient medical devices and telemedicine platforms
- Adopt sustainable practices in data center operations
- Engage with stakeholders to integrate sustainability considerations into digital health strategies

Specific actions:

- Implementing sustainable data center practices (e.g., using renewable energy, optimizing cooling systems)
- Developing eco-friendly medical devices with longer lifespans and easier repairability
- Optimizing telemedicine services to reduce unnecessary data transmission and energy use

2. Encouraging more environmentally conscious health care consumption

Promoting sustainable patient behavior in digital health can help minimize waste, conserve resources, and enable a more sustainable health care system.

What governments can do:

- Implement regulations to prevent greenwashing in digital health marketing
- Mandate transparency in the environmental impact of digital health services

- Collaborate with health care providers to raise awareness about sustainable digital health practices

What health care providers and technology companies can do:

- Provide patients with information on the environmental impact of different care options
- Offer incentives for choosing eco-friendly digital health services (e.g., lower-resolution telemedicine when appropriate)
- Develop tools to help patients track and reduce their health care-related carbon footprint

3. Improving the evidence base for informed policymaking

To make informed policy decisions and set realistic targets, stakeholders require reliable evidence on the environmental impact of digital health.

What governments can do:

- Establish mechanisms to collect data on the environmental impact of digital health services
- Require digital health companies to disclose information on their sustainability performance
- Fund research into innovative, sustainable digital health solutions

What international organizations can do:

- Advance understanding of the environmental impact of digital health through comprehensive research
- Facilitate collaboration among academia, industry, and policymakers to share data and best practices
- Foster partnerships to drive investment in environmentally sustainable digital health innovations

By implementing these recommendations, we can work toward a digital health future that truly embodies the principle of "First, do no harm"—not just for individual patients, but for our planet as a whole. This approach ensures that as we leverage technology to improve health care outcomes, we also minimize the environmental impact of these innovations, creating a sustainable health care system for future generations.

Chapter 7

Toward Environmentally Sustainable Digital Health that Works for Inclusive Health Care

7.1 Introduction

This chapter addresses the policy challenge of fostering environmentally sustainable digital health solutions that work for inclusive health care development. It emphasizes that policy responses at the national, regional, and international levels are more likely to succeed if they reflect the involvement of all stakeholders and holistically address digital health, socioeconomic, and environmental goals across the entire lifecycle of medical devices and health IT infrastructure.

Government strategies to mitigate greenhouse gas emissions, conserve resources, and reduce waste generation in health care should pay adequate attention to the environmental footprint of digital health technologies. Simultaneously, they should consider how these technologies can offer solutions to both health and environmental concerns.

Given the asymmetrical distribution of capabilities and resources in global health care, development partners are called upon to offer adequate support to low-income countries. This support should aim to strengthen their ability to participate effectively in a more circular global digital health economy that is also environmentally sustainable.

Key areas of focus include the following:

- Integrating environmental sustainability into digital health policies and strategies
- Developing regulatory frameworks that promote the ecofriendly design of medical devices and health IT systems
- Encouraging the adoption of renewable energy sources in health care data centers
- Promoting circular economy principles in the digital health sector
- Addressing the digital divide in health care to ensure equitable access to sustainable digital health solutions
- Fostering international cooperation for knowledge sharing and technology transfer in sustainable digital health practices

By addressing these challenges, we can work toward a future where digital health technologies not only improve patient outcomes but also contribute to environmental sustainability. This approach embodies the core principle of "First, do no harm," extending it from individual patient care to the health of our planet.

The chapter will explore policy options, best practices, and case studies from around the world, providing a roadmap for policymakers, health care providers, and technology companies to create a more sustainable and inclusive digital health ecosystem.

7.2 The Need for a New Policy Mindset in Digital Health

This book has explored the relationship between digital health and environmental sustainability, from the perspective of health care delivery and development. We've aimed to envision a digital health economy that leads to both environmental sustainability and inclusive health care.

The relationship between digital health and environmental impact is bidirectional. While digital health technologies have a significant and growing environmental footprint, they also offer solutions to both health and environmental challenges. We have primarily focused on the direct environmental impacts of digital health technologies.

Achieving environmentally sustainable digital health requires government policies and decisions by health care providers, technology companies, and patients that help reduce unsustainable practices along the lifecycle of digital health technologies, including production, use, and end-of-life.

Digital health divides are still widening, and various environmental costs associated with health care digitalization continue to rise. The new and complex interplay between digital health, health care development, and environmental sustainability points to the need for integrated policy responses. These responses should help bridge digital health divides and ensure that technological progress contributes to health equity while respecting planetary boundaries.

At present, the world is not on track for achieving either inclusive health care or environmental sustainability. For change to become a reality, a shift in mindset is needed. "Business as usual" is not an option. Exponential growth in digital health technologies and the associated demand for resources cannot be sustained as the reality of a finite planet becomes increasingly evident.

The current linear economy model in health care, based on "extract, make, use, dispose" is exhausting its resources. This calls for a move toward a circular economy model based on the principles of reducing, reusing, and recycling—approaches that favor reduced consumption and greater material recovery in health care. Such a shift could also stimulate new economic activities and job opportunities in the health sector, supporting inclusive development.

Moving toward a circular digital health economy would require changes in patient behavior, health care provider practices, and business models, as envisaged in Sustainable Development Goal 3 (good health and well-being) and Goal 12 (responsible consumption and production).

This chapter explores actions by relevant stakeholders and options for policymaking to foster environmentally sustainable digital health that works for inclusive health care development.

We discuss the following:

- The case for integrated treatment of digital health, environmental sustainability, and inclusive health care development
- Achieving sustainable consumption and production in health care through a circular approach
- Preconditions and fundamentals for better policymaking in digital health
- Policy options at different levels and stages of the digital health technology lifecycle
- The role of international cooperation in achieving sustainable digital health

By addressing these areas, we can work toward a future where digital health technologies not only improve patient outcomes but also contribute to environmental sustainability and global health equity. This approach truly embodies the principle of "First, Do No Harm," extending it from individual patient care to the health of our planet and global populations.

7.3 Aligning Digital Health, Environmental Sustainability, and Inclusive Health Care

7.3.1 Complex and Interconnected Global Health Challenges

The health care sector is undergoing a profound transformation driven by two major forces: (1) the rapid progress in digital health technologies and (2) the urgent need to move toward environmental sustainability. These interrelated drivers are mutually reinforcing, with key implications for inclusive health care development. Given the strong interface between digital health and environmental sustainability, associated challenges need to be assessed and addressed in an integrated manner.

The growing urgency to tackle these challenges has not yet been matched by a sufficiently integrated approach toward an inclusive and environmentally sustainable digital health future.

In fact, trends reviewed in this book leave little room for optimism:

- Digital health divides continue to widen, exacerbating health inequities globally.
- The concentration of market power is growing in the digital health economy, further accentuated by increased reliance on AI in health care.
- The proliferation of medical devices and expansion of health IT infrastructure is increasing demand for raw materials, some of which are in scarce supply.
- Environmentally and socially unsustainable practices persist in the production of digital health technologies.
- The digital health sector is consuming increasing amounts of energy and water, contributing to GHG emissions and threatening water availability.
- E-waste from obsolete medical devices is growing, while levels of reuse, repair, and recycling remain insufficient.

- While digital health innovations improve health care access and quality, they may also contribute to unsustainable levels of health care consumption and negative environmental impacts.

A continuation of current trajectories is not consistent with the need to comply with "planetary health boundaries." As more people gain access to digital health technologies and emerging technologies like AI, IoT, and virtual reality in health care are still in their infancy, it becomes increasingly important to consider how to reduce the direct environmental footprint of the digital health sector.

To address these challenges, we need an integrated approach that

- bridges digital health divides to ensure equitable access to health care technologies
- promotes sustainable production and consumption of digital health technologies
- encourages circular economy principles in the health care technology sector
- leverages digital health solutions to address both health and environmental challenges
- ensures that the benefits of digital health innovations are equitably distributed globally

By aligning digital health advancements with environmental sustainability and inclusive health care goals, we can work toward a future where technology improves health outcomes without compromising the health of our planet. This integrated approach embodies the true spirit of "First, do no harm," extending our care from individual patients to global populations and the environment that sustains us all.

7.3.2 Toward a Holistic, Whole of Life Cycle, and Multi-Stakeholder Approach in Digital Health

Achieving environmentally sustainable digital health that works for inclusive health care requires international cooperation and engagement from many stakeholders. Digital health transformation and environmental sustainability need to be considered jointly and holistically to move health care toward the sustainable-development future envisaged in the UN's 2030 Agenda for Sustainable Development.

Shaping an environmentally sustainable digital health economy that is also inclusive is complex and requires consideration of several dimensions:

- Digital health can have both positive and negative environmental impacts. Sustainable digital health involves direct effects from the production and use of health technologies and indirect effects from changes in health care delivery and patient behavior.
- Impacts occur at all stages in the life cycle of medical devices and health IT infrastructure.
- Environmental challenges emerge from digital health, including resource extraction for medical devices, energy and water use in health data centers, and e-waste from obsolete medical equipment.

Addressing these challenges requires collaboration among diverse stakeholders:

- academia and civil society organizations contributing research on digital health's environmental impact
- governments and international organizations setting policies and regulations for sustainable digital health
- scientists and developers designing sustainable health technologies
- health care providers and businesses implementing sustainable practices
- patients whose choices affect the environmental impact of health care

Policy responses need to reflect perspectives from countries at all levels of development, considering varying health care needs and digital capabilities.

Multi-stakeholder engagement has become increasingly important in both health and environmental domains. Enabling necessary actions and policies along the digital health life cycle is a joint responsibility of all stakeholders and countries.

The objective should be to maximize digital health's positive contribution to sustainability and minimize its negative impacts while ensuring inclusive health care outcomes. This requires a new culture of sustainable digital health and changes in mindsets and behaviors, built on principles of sustainable consumption and production in health care based on a circular economy approach.

Uncertainties related to environmental challenges and the rapid evolution of health technologies will require all stakeholders to adjust to evolving circumstances. There's no time to waste—decisions taken in the next few years will profoundly affect the digital health economy and its environmental impact long into the future.

By adopting this holistic, life cycle–oriented, and multi-stakeholder approach, we can work toward a digital health future that truly embodies the principle of "First, do no harm"—not just for individual patients but also for our planet and global health equity.

7.3.3 Harnessing the Principle of Common but Differentiated Responsibilities in Digital Health

The 2030 Agenda for Sustainable Development committed the global community to ensuring that no one, and no country, is left behind in the pursuit of sustainable development. Currently, benefits and costs from digital health are asymmetrically distributed. Developed countries have gained much more from health care digitalization than most developing countries. Most of the added value created in the digital health economy is captured by developed and digitally advanced developing countries. They have also contributed far more to its environmental footprint.

Conversely, many of the costs related to this footprint are incurred in lower-income countries. Developing countries are often locations of mining operations for materials used in medical devices and the destination for e-waste from obsolete health technologies. They are also particularly vulnerable to the health impacts of climate change. There are risks that least-developed countries (LDCs), in particular, will fall farther behind in terms of inclusive digital health development and environmental welfare.

Policy responses will have to consider this unequal ecological exchange and the situation of countries that are only at an early stage of health care digitalization. For digital health to be inclusive and environmentally sustainable, it must provide opportunities for governments, health care providers, and citizens in developing countries to participate effectively in increasingly digitalized health care markets and global health initiatives.

While there is a need at the global level to reduce the overconsumption of digital health technologies, especially in developed countries, bridging the digital health divide and raising digitalization levels in health care above the social floor remain critical preconditions for achieving equitable health outcomes and prosperity.

Efforts to foster environmentally sustainable digital health need to recognize that health care systems differ in their characteristics and abilities to engage in and benefit from digital health. Countries at different levels of development do not have the same capacities to address the challenges of digital health and environmental sustainability. They also have specific health needs to fulfill to meet their development objectives.

This situation raises concerns for developing countries, including the following:

- Resource-rich developing countries often supply raw materials for health technologies but generate little domestic value addition while paying for imported digital health equipment and services.
- As digital health adoption grows in developing countries, the health data generated domestically may be monetized by international digital health platforms rather than by local health care providers.
- Digital health policies, regulations, and standards are often shaped by and for developed countries, and are potentially ill-suited to the needs and capabilities of low-income countries.
- The digital health divide between low-income and more advanced countries continues to widen.

The principle of "common but differentiated responsibilities" is highly relevant in digital health. It acknowledges that while all countries share a responsibility to address global health and environmental challenges, the extent and nature of that responsibility vary according to each country's past responsibilities, capabilities, and level of development.

Actions by relevant stakeholders and policymaking at all levels should be founded on this principle. The steps taken should factor in the digital health needs in less advanced economies and ways to achieve health equity and social welfare within the framework of the Sustainable Development Goals while considering the constraints that governments may face in implementing sustainable digital health policies.

By applying this principle to digital health, we can work toward a future where technological advancements in health care benefit all populations while minimizing environmental impact, truly embodying the ethos of "First, do no harm" on a global scale.

7.4 Fostering Sustainable Consumption and Production in Digital Health Care

The rapid digitalization of health care has brought unprecedented advancements in patient care, diagnostics, and treatment. However, it has also raised significant environmental concerns, highlighting the urgent need for sustainable consumption and production practices. As emphasized in the Global Resources Outlook 2024, "it is no longer a question of whether a transformation toward global sustainable resource consumption and production is necessary, but how to urgently make it happen" (UNEP and IRP, 2024).

7.4.1 Applying Sustainable Development Goals to Digital Health Care

The framework for sustainable consumption and production, adopted at the 2012 United Nations Conference on Sustainable Development (Rio+20) provides a foundation for addressing these challenges. While the Sustainable Development Goal 12 targets link sustainable practices to economic prosperity, social welfare, and human rights, they don't explicitly address digitalization. However, these principles can and should be applied to the digital health care context:

- Efficient use of resources in the production of medical devices and digital health tools
- Reduction of e-waste from obsolete medical equipment and devices
- Promotion of energy-efficient data centers for health information systems
- Development of sustainable supply chains for digital health products

Sustainable digitalization and sustainability by design should be at the core of any emerging global governance framework for digital health technologies (UNEP, 2023b). This approach inherently incorporates sustainable consumption and production principles. Health care stakeholders should proactively shape the digital future, balancing digital and non-digital approaches to achieve sufficiency and circularity, rather than simply maximizing the reach of digital innovation (Digitalization for Sustainability, 2022).

The environmental impact of digital health care depends significantly on the relationship between consumers (patients, health care providers) and producers (medical device manufacturers, health IT companies) of digital health products and infrastructure. The following are among the key stakeholders:

- Governments: They can enable, promote, incentivize, and regulate behaviors to encourage environmentally sustainable practices in health care technology.
- Health care providers: As primary consumers of digital health technologies, they can demand and adopt more sustainable solutions.
- Patients: They can make informed choices about their use of digital health services and devices, considering environmental impacts.
- Health IT companies: They should prioritize sustainable design, production, and disposal practices for their products and services.
- Medical device manufacturers: They need to embrace circular economy principles in their production processes.
- Civil society organizations: They can support sustainable practices through advocacy, education, and monitoring.

7.4.2 Fostering Sustainable Consumption of Digital Health Products

In the rapidly evolving landscape of digital health care, consumers of health-related ICT goods and services are diverse, with varying needs and priorities. The increasing adoption of digital health technologies has led to new patterns of consumption, driven by such factors as follows:

- improved access to health information and services
- convenience of telemedicine and remote monitoring

- proliferation of health and wellness apps
- growing market for wearable health devices

While these advancements offer significant benefits, they also contribute to increased consumption and potential environmental impacts. Consumer choices in digital health are influenced by several factors:

- Clinical efficacy: the primary concern for most health care consumers
- Cost and value: especially important in health care systems with out-of-pocket expenses
- Convenience and accessibility: the ease of using digital health solutions
- Data privacy and security: critical concerns in handling sensitive health information
- User experience and interface: particularly important for patient-facing technologies
- Integration with existing health care systems: compatibility with electronic health records
- Regulatory compliance: adherence to health data protection laws and medical device regulations

Beyond these practical considerations, consumer choices may also be influenced by perceptions of cutting-edge technology and the status associated with using the latest digital health tools.

While there's growing awareness of environmental issues, sustainability often takes a backseat to immediate health concerns and technological capabilities in digital health. These are among the key challenges:

- frequent upgrades of health-related devices and software
- e-waste from obsolete medical devices and wearables
- energy consumption of always-on health monitoring systems
- data centers' environmental impact from storing and processing health data

To foster more sustainable consumption of digital health products, several strategies can be employed:

Raising awareness

- Educate health care providers and patients about the environmental impact of digital health technologies.
- Provide clear information on the carbon footprint and lifecycle of digital health products.

Incentivizing sustainable choices

- Develop eco-labeling systems for digital health products.
- Offer financial incentives for choosing environmentally friendly options.

Extending product lifespan

- Promote modular design in medical devices for easy upgrades and repairs.
- Encourage software updates over hardware replacements when possible.

Circular economy principles

- Establish take-back programs for used medical devices and wearables.
- Develop refurbishment and recycling programs for health IT equipment.

Sustainable design

- Encourage the development of energy-efficient health monitoring devices.
- Promote the use of sustainable materials in medical device manufacturing.

Drawing from the broader idea of digital sufficiency, we can define "digital health sufficiency" as the optimal use of digital health technologies that balance clinical efficacy, patient experience, and environmental sustainability. This concept encompasses the following:

- Hardware sufficiency: Minimizing the number of devices required for effective health monitoring and care delivery.
- Software sufficiency: Optimizing health apps and systems to reduce unnecessary data traffic and processing.
- User sufficiency: Encouraging judicious use of digital health tools, avoiding overreliance on technology where traditional methods may suffice.
- Economic sufficiency: Promoting a health care economy that prioritizes value-based care and sustainable practices over purely profit-driven innovation.

Fostering sustainable consumption in digital health requires a collaborative effort:

- Health care providers: They can prioritize sustainable digital health solutions in their procurement processes.
- Patients: They can make informed choices about their use of digital health products and services.
- Health IT companies: They should incorporate sustainability principles into their product design and development.
- Policymakers: They can create regulations that incentivize sustainable practices in digital health.
- Health insurers: They can offer incentives for using sustainable digital health solutions.

As we embrace the potential of digital technologies to transform health care, we must also consider their environmental impact. By fostering sustainable consumption practices in digital health, we can ensure that our efforts to improve human health do not come at the cost of environmental health. This aligns with the core principle of "First, do no harm," extending it beyond individual patient care to encompass our broader responsibility to the planet.

7.4.3. Fostering Sustainable Production in Digital Health Care

The digital health sector, like much of the tech industry, has traditionally been driven by rapid innovation and market growth. This approach, while leading to significant advancements in health care delivery and patient outcomes, often overlooks potential environmental impacts. The following are among the key challenges:

- Frequent upgrades of medical devices and health IT infrastructure
- Short lifespans of digital health products
- Energy-intensive data centers for health information systems
- E-waste from obsolete medical equipment and devices

Digital health businesses face unique challenges and opportunities in adopting sustainable practices:

- Regulatory compliance: Strict medical device regulations can slow the pace of change but also provide opportunities for integrating sustainability requirements.
- Data-driven revenue models: Many digital health platforms rely on gathering and analyzing patient data, which can incentivize excessive data collection and storage.
- Interoperability requirements: The need for systems to work together across health care providers can lead to resistance to change.
- Patient safety priorities: The primary focus on patient safety and clinical efficacy can sometimes overshadow environmental considerations.

To foster more sustainable production in digital health care, several strategies can be employed:

Sustainable design principles

- Incorporate environmental considerations into the design phase of digital health products.
- Develop modular medical devices to facilitate repairs, upgrades, and recycling.
- Design software and AI algorithms with energy efficiency in mind.

Lifecycle assessments

- Conduct comprehensive environmental impact assessments for digital health products and services.
- Consider the entire supply chain, from raw material sourcing to end-of-life disposal.

Transparency and reporting

- Collect and report detailed information on the environmental performance of digital health products.
- Implement independent scrutiny to prevent greenwashing and ensure accurate reporting.

Collaboration and resource optimization

- Encourage partnerships within the health care industry to minimize resource use.
- Optimize the use of data centers and networks, potentially through shared infrastructure.

Circular economy in health care

- Develop robust systems for the reuse and recycling of medical devices and IT equipment.

- Implement take-back programs for obsolete health tech products.

Standard-setting bodies in health care technology should prioritize environmental sustainability alongside technical efficiency and patient safety. This could include the following:

- Developing eco-design standards for medical devices
- Creating energy efficiency benchmarks for health IT systems
- Establishing guidelines for sustainable data management in health care

To encourage sustainable innovation in digital health, several approaches can be considered:

- Provide funding and grants for research into sustainable health technologies
- Offer tax incentives for companies that meet specific sustainability targets
- Implement sustainability criteria in public procurement of health technologies

Given the concentration of market power in the digital health sector, actions taken by leading companies can have significant ripple effects:

- Improvements in the energy efficiency of major health IT platforms can impact the entire health care ecosystem.
- Sustainable practices adopted by large medical device manufacturers can influence their entire supply chain.

Adopting sustainable practices can offer several benefits to digital health companies:

- Reduced production costs through resource efficiency
- New revenue streams from repair and refurbishment services
- Enhanced brand reputation and customer loyalty
- Improved resilience to environmental regulations and resource scarcity

Fostering sustainable production in digital health care requires a paradigm shift from a model focused solely on rapid innovation and market growth to one that balances clinical efficacy, economic viability, and environmental sustainability. By integrating sustainability into the core of digital health innovation, we can ensure that our efforts to improve human health through technology do not come at the cost of environmental health.

7.4 Moving Toward Circularity in Digital Health Care

The concept of a circular economy offers a sustainable foundation for business models in digital health care, focusing on enhancing the longevity, utilization, and overall lifetime of medical devices and health IT products. By prioritizing product life extension strategies such as maintenance, repair, refurbishing, and recycling, the health care sector can reduce the need for new products and the corresponding extraction of raw materials, thereby minimizing waste and environmental impact.

Adopting circular economy principles in digital health care can create valuable opportunities for economic growth and job creation while contributing to sustainable development. The business case for circularity in health care technology includes:

- Cost reduction: Extending the life of medical devices and IT equipment, which can lower health care providers' capital expenditures
- Resource security: Reducing dependence on scarce materials used in electronic components
- Innovation opportunities: Developing new technologies and services around repair, refurbishment, and recycling of medical devices
- Regulatory compliance: Meeting increasingly stringent environmental regulations in the health care sector
- Brand enhancement: Improving reputation among environmentally conscious patients and health care professionals

To enable a more environmentally sustainable digital health care ecosystem, circularity needs to be factored in at every stage of the product lifecycle:

Design and innovation

- Develop modular medical devices that are easy to repair and upgrade.
- Design health IT systems with long-term compatibility and scalability in mind.
- Create software that can run efficiently on older hardware to extend device lifespans.

Manufacturing

- Use recycled materials in the production of medical devices where possible.
- Implement lean manufacturing processes to minimize waste.
- Prioritize the use of non-toxic, recyclable materials in medical technology.

Use and maintenance

- Provide comprehensive maintenance services to extend the life of medical equipment.
- Offer software updates to improve functionality without hardware replacement.
- Implement predictive maintenance using AI to prevent equipment failures.

End-of-life management

- Establish take-back programs for obsolete medical devices and IT equipment.
- Develop specialized recycling processes for medical technology.
- Refurbish and redeploy older equipment to health care facilities in underserved areas.

Moving toward a circular model in digital health care can lead to multiple benefits:

- Environmental impact reduction: Minimizing e-waste and reducing the demand for raw materials
- Improved resource efficiency: Optimizing the use of scarce resources in medical technology
- Cost savings: Lowering the total cost of ownership for health care providers through extended product lifespans
- Innovation stimulation: Encouraging the development of more sustainable health care technologies
- Job creation: Generating new roles in repair, refurbishment, and recycling of medical technology

While the benefits are significant, implementing circularity in digital health care faces unique challenges:

- Regulatory compliance: Ensuring that refurbished medical devices meet stringent safety standards
- Data security: Addressing concerns about patient data when repurposing or recycling health IT equipment
- Technological obsolescence: Balancing the need for the latest medical innovations with sustainability goals
- Initial costs: Overcoming the upfront investments required to transition to circular models

Achieving greater circularity in digital health care requires concerted action from all stakeholders:

- Health care providers: Prioritize procurement of sustainable and repairable medical technology.
- Medical device manufacturers: Design for longevity, repairability, and recyclability.
- Health IT companies: Develop software that can run efficiently on older hardware.

- Policymakers: Create regulations that incentivize circular practices in health care technology.
- Patients: Advocate for sustainable practices in health care delivery.

Moving toward circularity in digital health care represents a paradigm shift in how we approach medical technology and health IT systems. By embracing circular economy principles, the health care sector can significantly reduce its environmental footprint while potentially improving access to medical technology through cost reductions and innovative reuse strategies. This approach aligns perfectly with the ethos of "First, do no harm," extending it beyond patient care to encompass environmental stewardship. As we continue to advance digital health care, circularity offers a path to ensure that our efforts to improve human health do not come at the cost of planetary health.

Chapter 8

Policy Options for Environmentally Sustainable Digital Development

8.1 Introduction

Achieving environmentally sustainable digitalization that supports inclusive development requires an integrated, holistic approach to policymaking. This chapter provides an overview of key policy options and considerations for governments and other stakeholders.

Given the complex, interdisciplinary nature of the issues involved, policies need to address the entire life cycle of digital technologies—from mineral extraction and manufacturing, through usage, to end-of-life disposal, and recycling. Additionally, a multi-stakeholder approach is crucial, involving governments, businesses, civil society, and international organizations.

These are among the key policy areas to consider:

- integrating digital and environmental sustainability strategies
- managing the extraction and use of critical minerals
- promoting energy efficiency and renewable energy use in ICT
- extending product lifespans and enabling repairs

- facilitating e-waste collection and recycling
- fostering circular economy practices
- supporting sustainable consumption behaviors

The appropriate mix of policy instruments will vary based on national contexts, but it may include the following:

- legislation and regulations (e.g., on e-waste, energy efficiency standards)
- economic incentives (e.g., tax breaks for green ICT, fees on nonrecyclable electronics)
- information provision and awareness campaigns
- public procurement policies prioritizing sustainable ICT
- support for R&D on green digital technologies
- capacity-building initiatives, especially in developing countries

Integrating Digital and Environmental Strategies

To achieve policy coherence, governments should update and integrate their digitalization and environmental sustainability strategies as part of comprehensive national development plans.

Examples of integrated approaches:

- France's Interministerial Mission for Eco-Responsible Digitalization
- Germany's Digital Policy Agenda for the Environment
- The European Union's linking of digital transition and Green Deal policies
- South Korea's alignment of green ICT strategy with emissions reduction targets

Coordinated strategies should draw on expertise from across government ministries as well as external stakeholders. The following are among the key elements:

- setting targets for reducing the environmental footprint of the ICT sector

- policies to extend product lifespans and combat planned obsolescence
- promoting energy-efficient data centers and networks
- supporting the development of digital solutions for environmental challenges
- building digital and environmental skills

Managing Critical Minerals

The rising demand for minerals needed for digital technologies and low-carbon solutions requires careful policy attention.

The following are among the key considerations:

- ensuring sustainable and ethical mining practices
- promoting recycling and urban mining to reduce primary extraction
- developing substitutes for scarce minerals
- supporting developing countries in capturing more value from mineral resources
- international cooperation on mineral governance and supply chain transparency

Promoting Sustainable Consumption and Production

Policies are needed to shift both business models and consumer behaviors toward sustainability.

For businesses

- extended producer responsibility schemes
- eco-design requirements for electronics
- mandatory repairability standards
- transparency on environmental impacts

For consumers

- awareness campaigns on sustainable electronic use
- incentives for device repair and recycling
- tools to compare products' environmental footprints
- support for product-as-a-service business models

Fostering a Circular Digital Economy

Transitioning to a more circular model for electronics and ICT infrastructure requires the following:

- policies to extend product lifespans (right to repair, modular design)
- improved collection and recycling systems for e-waste
- standards and incentives for using recycled materials in new products
- support for refurbishment and remanufacturing industries
- trade policies that enable circular economy practices

International Cooperation

Given the global nature of digital technology supply chains and environmental challenges, strengthened international cooperation is essential.

The following are among the priority areas:

- developing harmonized standards and metrics on ICT sustainability
- technology transfer and capacity building for developing countries
- coordinated approaches to managing critical mineral supply chains
- cooperation in tackling the illegal trade in e-waste
- integrating environmental considerations into digital trade agreements

Policy Coherence and Implementation

To be effective, policies must be coherent across different domains and levels of governance.

The following are among the key success factors:

- whole-of-government approaches to align digital, environmental, and development policies
- stakeholder engagement in policy design and implementation
- strengthened data collection and impact assessment capabilities
- flexible, adaptive policymaking to keep pace with technological change
- adequate resources for enforcement and monitoring

While there is no one-size-fits-all approach, all countries need to develop integrated policy frameworks to harness digital technologies for sustainable development. Policies should aim to maximize the environmental and social benefits of digitalization while minimizing negative impacts across the technology lifecycle.

International cooperation and support for developing countries will be crucial to ensure an inclusive global transition to sustainable digital development. With the right policies and multi-stakeholder collaboration, digitalization can become a powerful enabler of environmental sustainability and inclusive economic progress.

Conclusion

As we conclude our exploration of the complex intersection between health care digitalization and environmental sustainability, it is clear that the health care sector stands at a critical juncture. The rapid adoption of AI and digital technologies offers unprecedented opportunities to enhance patient care, improve health outcomes, and increase access to health services. However, these advancements come with significant environmental implications that we can no longer afford to ignore.

Throughout this book, we have examined the health care sector's substantial climate footprint and the urgent need for action to mitigate its environmental impact. We have also delved into the transformative potential of digital health technologies and their ability to both address and exacerbate environmental challenges. As we chart a path forward, several key themes emerge:

- Holistic Approach to Innovation

The health care sector must adopt a holistic approach to innovation that considers both the benefits and environmental costs of new technologies. This means evaluating the entire lifecycle of digital health products and systems, from raw material extraction to end-of-life disposal. By integrating environmental considerations into the design and implementation of digital health solutions, we can maximize their positive impact while minimizing their ecological footprint.

- Balancing Progress and Sustainability

As we strive to improve health care delivery and outcomes through digitalization, we must simultaneously work to reduce the sector's overall environmental impact. This delicate balance requires careful planning, innovative thinking, and a commitment to sustainability at all levels of health care organizations. It also necessitates collaboration among health care providers, technology developers, policymakers, and environmental experts to create solutions that advance both health and environmental goals.

- Leveraging Technology for Environmental Benefits

While digital technologies can contribute to environmental challenges, they also offer powerful tools for addressing them. From AI-driven energy management systems in hospitals to telemedicine platforms that reduce travel-related emissions, digital solutions can play a crucial role in making health care more environmentally sustainable. The key lies in strategically deploying these technologies to maximize their positive environmental impact.

- Addressing Global Health Inequities

As we pursue a more sustainable digital health care future, we must remain mindful of global health inequities. The transition to digital health technologies should not exacerbate existing disparities but, rather, serve as a means to bridge them. This requires careful consideration of how digital solutions are developed, implemented, and accessed across different regions and populations.

- Cultivating a Culture of Sustainability

Building a sustainable health care future requires more than just technological solutions; it demands a fundamental shift in mindset across the entire health care ecosystem. From medical education to organizational policies, we must cultivate a culture that values environmental sustainability as integral to the mission of health care.

- Continuous Learning and Adaptation

The field of digital health is rapidly evolving, as is our understanding of environmental sustainability. Health care organizations must commit to continuous learning and adaptation, staying abreast of new technologies and sustainability practices to ensure they are always at the forefront of environmentally responsible health care delivery.

- Policy and Regulatory Framework

Achieving a sustainable digital health care future will require supportive policy and regulatory frameworks. Governments and international bodies must work to create incentives for sustainable practices in health care, set standards for the environmental performance of digital health technologies, and facilitate the sharing of best practices across borders.

As we look to the future, it is clear that the health care sector has both a responsibility and an opportunity to lead in the fight against climate change. By embracing sustainable digitalization, we can create a health care system that not only provides excellent care but also protects and nurtures the environment that sustains us all.

The journey toward a sustainable digital health care future will not be easy. It will require dedication, innovation, and collaboration on an unprecedented scale. However, the stakes could not be higher. The health of our patients and the health of our planet are inextricably linked, and it is our duty as health care providers to safeguard both.

As we move forward, let us remember that every decision we make in implementing digital health technologies has the potential to impact both human and planetary health. By staying true to our fundamental principle of "First, do no harm" and extending it to encompass environmental considerations, we can build a health care system that truly serves the well-being of all.

The future of health care lies not just in technological advancement but also in sustainable innovation that respects the delicate balance of our ecosystem. It is time for the health care sector to take the lead in demonstrating how we can harness the power of technology to heal not just individuals but also our entire planet. The path ahead is challenging, but with commitment, creativity, and collaboration, we can create a digital health care future that is both cutting-edge and sustainable, serving as a model for other sectors and generations to come.

About the Author

Dr. Rubin Pillay is a distinguished physician, researcher, and thought leader in the fields of health care innovation and sustainability. With a medical degree (MD) and a PhD, he has dedicated his career to advancing the intersection of health care and technology, focusing on how digital innovations can improve patient outcomes while addressing pressing environmental challenges.

Dr. Pillay has extensive experience in health care administration and policy, having held leadership positions in various health care organizations. His work emphasizes the importance of integrating sustainable practices within health care systems to mitigate their environmental impact. He is a passionate advocate for leveraging artificial intelligence (AI) and digital technologies to enhance the efficiency and effectiveness of health care delivery while ensuring that these advancements do not compromise the health of our planet.

In addition to his clinical practice, Dr. Pillay is an accomplished researcher, contributing to numerous publications on topics related to digital health, climate change, and health equity. He frequently speaks at national and international conferences, sharing his insights on the future of health care in an increasingly digital world.

Through *First, Do No Harm: Building a Sustainable Health Care Future with AI and Digital Technologies*, Dr. Pillay aims to inspire health care professionals, policymakers, and technologists to embrace a holistic approach to digitalization—one that prioritizes both health outcomes and environmental sustainability. His vision is for a future where health care not only heals individuals but also protects the planet for generations to come.

www.ingramcontent.com/pod-product-compliance
Lightning Source LLC
Chambersburg PA
CBHW020420220526
45464CB00002B/508